Praise for Claudio Mochi's *Beyond the Clouds*

"What an amazing way to learn about and explore the world of good practice in crisis intervention! This immersive, enchanting book sucked me in to Claudio Mochi's professional (and many times personal) world—his thoughts, experiences, feelings, reactions, knowledge, and wisdom. With Mochi's poetic writing, engaging metaphors, intriguing quotes, descriptions of real-life crisis situations, and a practical process/intervention model, this book will stimulate your brain, evoke your emotions, and inspire your actions."

Terry Kottman, Ph.D., RPT-S, LMHC, NCC

Founder and Director League of Extraordinary Adlerian Play Therapists

"Midway through Claudio Mochi's enthralling text, he quotes Korzybski who said 'The map is not the territory.' Though perhaps not the actual territory, I cannot imagine a better map than *Beyond the Clouds*. As thrilling as an adventure novel, as informative as the thickest textbook, and as personal and moving as the most intimate memoir, Mochi gives us a map and invites us on the journey to understand at the deepest level what it is to intervene in crisis situations with intention, care, and humility. Read it twice! I did."

Jeff Ashby, PhD, ABPP, RPT-S

Professor, Counseling Psychology

Director, Play Therapy Training Institute

Co-Director, Center for the Study of Stress, Trauma, and Resilience, Georgia State University

"Mochi is a master storyteller who beautifully blends science and theory with his vast experience as he takes us on his personal journey working in crises intervention. In this highly accessible volume, enhanced by his use of metaphor and story, Mochi outlines core dimensions of best practices in crises intervention. A must read—I could not put it down!"

—Sue C. Bratton, PhD, LPC-S, RPT-S, Professor Emerita and Director Emerita, Center for Play Therapy, University of North Texas.

Beyond the Clouds is a beautiful gift, an inspiration, and a call to action. The premise of pausing long enough to process the reciprocity between those of us who want to be of service and those who are recipients, is profound. Claudio is purposeful in his work and he shares what he has learned with great generosity and humility. It transported me and I highly recommend!"

—Eliana Gil, Ph.D., Gil Institute for Trauma Recovery & Education. Fairfax, Virginia.

Beyond the Clouds

An Autoethnographic Research
Exploring Good Practice in Crisis Settings

Claudio Mochi

Loving Healing Press

Ann Arbor, MI

Beyond the Clouds: An Autoethnographic Research Exploring Good Practice in Crisis Settings

ISBN 978-1-61599-672-8 paperback
ISBN 978-1-61599-673-5 hardcover
ISBN 978-1-61599-674-2 eBook

Published by
Loving Healing Press   www.LHPress.com
5145 Pontiac Trail   info@LHPress.com
Ann Arbor, MI 48105

Tollfree 888-761-6268
FAX 734-663-686`

This writing is dedicated to my father who taught me a lot just by "going on a cruise."

Contents

Table of Figures

Acknowledgments

I thank my mom, who during our walks helped me to complete many of the thoughts that have given rise to some of these pages. I thank her for always encouraging me to follow my own path, even when it would have been convenient and comforting for her to have me close by.

I owe all the colleagues with whom I have worked a huge thank you for the many personal and professional insights that have helped me to grow.

I express my deep gratitude to Mr. Mustafa on behalf of all those affected by exceptional circumstances. Mr. Mustafa has done me the honor of sharing his terrible past with me, showing me how it is possible to move forward and write new chapters of our life even in the most tragic circumstances. In my heart, his teaching, and that of so many other *super*vivors, still goes beyond what I am able to put into words at the moment.

I would like to thank Victor Volkman for believing in this project from the start and for the opportunity he has given me to share this journey through the clouds with the reader.

There is my name on the cover of this book, but in truth every single word and concept was discussed with and reviewed by my life and working partner Isabella Cassina.

Isabella is not only a continuous source of motivation, but she has been a guide in this process. To me, Isabella is both Beatrice and Virgil, especially in this book. Not only we have been working side by side for years in the co-construction of various types of projects, but in this journey she has helped me to always proceed *diagonally*, upward and forward. I was able to elaborate and advance in this work through her questions, reflections and editing work.

Beyond the Clouds could not be the same without her creations. The figures and drawings are hers, as well as a number of activities that have been included, but I will not mention them here so as not to reveal anything in advance to the reader.

Introduction

This book aims to explore the constituent elements of good practice in crisis intervention. It is developed through a metaphorical journey across the clouds, toward a clear sky for descending to the destination.

The approach used is an introspective investigation in which the "clouds" represent the implicit experiences of the author; the "clear sky" is the moment for reflection and understanding, where implicit knowledge becomes explicit; and the descent is the moment when enriched experience and new knowledge are integrated in our autobiographical story and can be "translated into practice."

This research parallels the right-left-right progression described in the last chapter and emphasizes the fundamental role of three elements: the safe space and the use of symbols that allow individuals contact with implicit experiences, writing as a tool to focus and analyze relevant past experiences, and the metaphor as a means to reintegrate the experience.

Crises are complex, often chaotic, and occur within rapidly changing contexts. Being an "added value" requires the professional in the field to balance the need to rely on clear conceptual maps and the ability to be flexible. In this challenging work of adaptation, an essential reference is provided by the core dimensions of good practice: respect, effectiveness and safety, which offer a solid starting point to build the intervention.

Adapting the maps to the territory and translating knowledge and experience into practice are not automatic processes; they are instead the result of an intentional and well-cultivated exercise.

Consequently, good practice for professionals does not require just the comprehension of the different dimensions, but needs to be rooted in preparation that includes regular introspective research and self-care.

1   Take Off

Last journal entry of the day (22.01 GMT-5): my name is Claudio, I am a psychologist specializing in disaster mental health interventions. During the twenty-plus hours of air travel today I learned a lot and, more than ever, I feel being the author of my own story. In eleven hours, I will start training my colleagues in dealing with the psychological impact of the earthquake that hit the island and together we will build a crisis intervention.

Everything is ready and I do not feel like sleeping now. On the journey to this massive disaster, I realized something very important: I have been working in crises all over the world, but have done insufficient work on my own internal travel. Even though it is late and tomorrow will be a long and intense day, I want to write down every detail of this experience "beyond the clouds" and learn from it. I cannot procrastinate, not after today. Moreover it won't be difficult, it's all still very vivid and present in my mind. In fact, it will help me sleep better. I'll just have to go through my thoughts from the moment I sat in the airplane and add what I haven't already jotted down in my journal.

Maybe one day I will also share this writing. I think it might be interesting for colleagues working in similar contexts and those "explorers" and "would-be explorers" who do not give up their search, even in "poor visibility conditions."

Twenty-plus hours before...

I made it. No crazy rush with full bags, extra layers of clothing nor sweat-soaked t-shirts. Nothing to feel ashamed of so far. We will see—some spots might appear on my clothes after I have eaten.

My bag is overfilled as usual, and it does not allow me much space for the legs. I probably won't need everything I'd packed, but you never know. Good to sit near the window, on the wings "of course," but still, I can see outside. I certainly won't miss the feeling of being in the way between a person and his toileting needs. The guy next to me looks calm. For once, I am also relaxed and hope nobody from the row behind me will play with my seat for the next twelve hours.

The airplane is moving and I cannot help to think, what has happened where I am headed and what I am going to find there. Even though I have been in similar circumstances before, sometimes it is difficult to realize that behind those dramatic images on the TV are real stories of pain, loss and despair. I must prepare myself before arriving, but I do not like watching news reports. What happened is so deep, powerful and inconceivable. Yes, I guess "inconceivable" is the right term. Cognitively, I do not think we can really grasp what actually happens when everything we longed for, loved and built disappears, when the whole life we were attached to is destroyed in a few moments. How can we make our minds fathom this?

I received a document from our local partner; it is brief but full of information. Let me see, they are not sure about the number of casualties. Anyway, does it really matter how extended the destruction is? In most cases the people I am going to meet have lost almost everything. If you are hit by a tragedy, does it truly matter for you that other thousands of people had a "similar" tragedy?

Twenty years ago, while assessing a possible partnership with me, I remember the psychiatrist in Iran asking: "How many people died where you worked the last time?" I do not recall his name, but I can still see his face when I said: "Thirty." I guess he was weighing my experience and my tolerance to stress. We cooperated eventually, but I was offended by his reaction to my answer, because he implied that the suffering of thirty families was a less serious situation. I would have liked to tell him how the life of an entire village was destroyed, a whole region upset and an entire nation touched by that event. By judging from his coldness to the subject, I thought he, along the way, had lost something by witnessing too much suffering, or maybe power and responsibilities might have unbalanced him.

So much time has passed since our exchange and I now understand that basically he was missing a key aspect in that conversation: the process. If a professional is not part of a structure and a process, he cannot be supportive to one, twenty-eight or one thousand persons. If I were he, today I would have probably asked: "Which kind of process are you suggesting? What is your experience in this regard?" It is curious how adding a line to this story cheered me up a little.

The guy next to me on the airplane seems absorbed in his thoughts. Slowly we taxi on the runway and are now in the queue for taking off. It is a beautiful, sunny day. This time I will not skip a season or two and the grass will still be green when I return home.

I usually feel nostalgic at this point, but not this time. Maybe I am getting more organized. I did not have to rush for last minute errands. I do not even feel tired. There is such diversity in the world: some people get very tense when the airplane takes off; for me, it is usually the moment I begin to feel more relaxed. The guy close to me also seems very composed. No envy for him sitting in the middle. The fact I am not feeling tired could also be another sign that I paced myself better for this departure. Let me write this point down. Here is my journal, my best friend in these situations. *Maybe, after almost twenty years, I have learned something.*[1] This is a good starting point for my writing.

Since Isabella and I have started working together, this is the first time I have left alone. Perhaps this is why I am having such a rush of past memories. She will reach me in a few days but, if she were here, she would probably say, "Is this another Memory Day of yours?" I like her irony, she always makes me smile with this joke. Am I

---

[1] The parts of the text written in italics correspond to what the author of this research writes in his "copybook." they include personal reflections, notes and quotes for his next training program for local professionals in a crisis setting.

becoming like the fictional character, *Mr. Higgins*[2]? I do not like this idea, because although he is charming in his own way, every time he starts telling a story, people vanish! I always wanted to be more like *Magnum*. Anyway, I guess it makes sense having all these memories floating around today. This recalling is most probably a way to get mentally ready for the situation I will soon face.

Some call it a "mission." Well, it is not. It is a profession and as such it requires specific preparation and relevant experience (Inter-Agency Standing Committee, 2007, p.73) and a structure where the expertise can be provided. Most importantly, a "mission" for me is something you dedicate completely with no restraint, risking everything. On the contrary, in any profession, you have to balance your working commitment with other components of life.

I can hear my friend Paolo's words when he talks about Greek architecture: "Beauty is in the perfection of the proportions of the different elements. Humans are wired to appreciate and enjoy good proportions." I believe he is right and proportions are relevant also for any professional. For instance, how much time and energy to dedicate to different aspects such as personal needs, family, actual working practice, study, research, self-care, and professional growth? There is so much to balance for a worker in crisis scenarios. I like the idea Isabella and I formulated for a conference in Australia (Mochi, 2017). It is about the characters from *The Wizard of Oz*[3] following the Yellow Brick Road. Let me figure out how it was and prepare a note card[4]:

---

[2] Mr. Higgins and Thomas Magnum are fictional characters of the 1980s American drama television series *Magnum P.I.*

[3] *The Wizard of Oz* (1939) is an American musical fantasy film. The story is about a girl named Dorothy and her dog, Toto, who, after a cyclone, find themselves in the Land of Oz Following the Yellow Brick Road to reach the Emerald City and to meet the Wizard, they encounter three characters: a Scarecrow in search of a brain, a Tin Man that longs for a heart, and a Lion that would like courage.

[4] The gray boxes inserted all along the pages represent the "note cards" created by the author as a support for the forthcoming training.

Dorothy: capability for community involvement and to connect with existing resources.

Toto: positive energy and playfulness.

Scarecrow: specific expertise, focus and common sense.

Tin Man: heart to connect with people, attune to their needs, ability to provide caring and nourishing experiences.

Lion: confidence in ability and experience, the ability to provide a calm and reassuring presence.

It is extremely important to have all members along the "road," and their presence needs to be proportionate to the situation. Thinking in these terms, the psychiatrist I'd recalled before was accompanied by the Lion and the Scarecrow: confident expertise. They dominated the scene, to me appearing to leave the other characters mostly in the shade. A constructive activity to suggest at some point of my training could be answering the following questions: "How would I assess myself in those realms in my work? What is dominant at the moment and what is the area where I feel I would like to improve?" The Yellow Brick Road analogy as intended here fits well in a crisis context, but I also see how it could make sense in private practice. I guess any individual in the helping professions should find the appropriate companions for his path and work on the right proportions.

So here I am, in the airplane, getting prepared for work with my silent Memory Day. Looking outside the window, I realize I overcame the internal debate on the relevance and value of my work. Psychological intervention post-disaster is such a specific field that deals with profound wounds, irremediable losses, offering such intangible support. The value of this kind of intervention is not always understood, and often in the field I have to explain what our work is about. I remember a heart surgeon telling me: "We save children's lives. What do *you* do instead?" She could definitely talk straight. "We are there immediately after that, trying to help children to have better lives" (this was my direct answer) "because by improving their emotional wellbeing, fostering their development and enhancing specific skills, we can help children to improve the quality of their lives." In that moment I noticed a softening of her stony face. The most important thing a human can do is definitely to save another person's life. Immediately after that, the best we can do is to help this person to enjoy and improve his life. I believe that a genuine group and a community effort have tremendous potential in impacting the quality of life even in the most distressing situations. It is interesting how, a few years later, we introduced a similar concept in our work, using as theoretical reference, "The person-centered approach in the human development perspective," which has the objective of supporting individuals in expanding their capabilities in order to have more opportunities and life choices (United Nations Development Programme, 2016, p.25).

Maureen[5] was right: therapists have to undertake their own personal therapy. At the time, I thought it should not be an obligation because not everybody has issues. Nowadays, I realize that personal therapy can help any process to be smoother: emotions, doubts, physical sensations can be easier connected with thoughts, we can expand our perspectives, inform our decisions and plans. Here I am, getting more clarity in the middle of the clouds.

---

[5] "Maureen" is the invented name for a real professional who is the director of a psychotherapy training center. In several meetings dedicated to build international training standards, she advocated the need for therapists to undertake their own personal therapy.

2   In the Clouds

It is a good moment to eat my sandwich. Other passengers are having their meal and I can finally taste my Parma ham even if I question its authenticity. I did not want to look spoiled to my neighbor so I just said I am on a diet. From his facial expression, I think he had no difficulty believing me. Damn, now I have to be consistent for the rest of the journey. It took me "only" thirty years to recognize my need and to adjust to it. Two Euros and three minutes of preparation were enough to make my journey nicer. I guess I am used to going with the "automatic pilot" more than I expected. The funny thing is that, at this moment, we are surely flying on automatic pilot, but two professionals ensure that the system follows the plan.

Cloud after cloud, the flow of thoughts and feelings is increasing and swarming in my mind. It is like they were waiting for me along the way. Disorienting and destabilizing travel companions, I would really like to have you quiet and still but I cannot control you and, also if I did, it would require quite some focus and time to sort all this material out. I am sure whatever process I could start, the Scarecrow, the Tin Man and the Lion would be helpful. This is a bizarre idea: "Hey guys, come here please! I need you." As weird as it may sound, the idea to have helpers can work. I have to tell Isabella about this. It is not that absurd after all, because it is a way to activate cortical modulation[6] (Perry, 1997, p.129).

---

[6] Cortical Modulation is the capacity of the more complex limbic, sub-cortical and cortical areas to modulate, moderate and "control" the more primitive and "reactive" lower portions of the brain (Perry 1997).

Following Siegel's house metaphor (Siegel and Bryson, 2016, pp. 21-2), when I called on the company of Oz I started to connect the two floors of my "house." The primitive downstairs brain perceived something threatening and started to react. This is where my unclear and uncomfortable body sensations and feelings come from. The moment I think of the Scarecrow, the Lion and the Tin Man, I invite the upstairs part of the brain to join. As the responsible and rational component, this upper part seeks to understand what is going on and tries to put some order into chaos. Maybe it sounds a little crazy, but it makes sense and it is a possibility. There is more to it. Just playing with these ideas, I realized that I have helpers with me. In this moment and during the work that I am going to do, I will have by my side the knowledge and the skills I developed, the confidence I gained in my experience, and the connection with my own feelings.

Dear neighbor, you do not have any idea how weird the thoughts of psychologists can be. Anyway, analogies are very helpful to anchor my strategies. Now that my company of Oz is activated, I can go back to the clouds. Let me write a note on what this cloud-iness is all about: *What will happen at the moment I arrive there? Will I be able to cooperate with this organization and to work with the local team? Will I find a way to connect with the survivors? How will I deal with unrealistic expectations? Will I have enough time? Am I adding value?* I wonder if and how this work will improve the quality of somebody's life.

I believe those whirling thoughts are part of the deed, provoking both anxiety and good reflections. I am also aware that I do not know what will happen and how this experience is going to affect me, but I can predict that it will. Luckily, other people's pain, helplessness and deprivation do not leave us indifferent. I think of the project in Palestine. What we built back then became a model for other projects. And yet, doing my best and working with excellent professionals still left a great sense of helplessness and lack of control in me. The more I distanced myself from the context, the deeper were my feelings. At the time, I did not know how to make sense of certain circumstances and how to describe the complex stories I was witnessing. Even now, I struggle to express in words the extent of my lived human and professional experiences. Months after the end of my job, I realized the mess of sensations and doubts I had. My self-care routine, the supervision and the journal were not enough to help me to find order and meaning. I needed more structure and more clarity to recognize what I was carrying inside. In that moment, I resolved to write an article.

As in undertaking a research project, I had to state my research questions on paper, and embedded doubts to force me to a deeper investigation and to find possible scientific answers. I had to grab two of the biggest clouds around myself, the stormy ones. Unintentionally, the selection of the most hurtful feelings and confusing doubts paid off. Also, taking time to write paid off. Only a handful of people read it, but it was a health matter; I did not care about publishing, sharing, showing or teaching. I cared about my need to find meanings, answers or at least to give a proper space to my doubts. It is amazing how much the words of Bochner (SMCBGSU, 2016) resonate with my experience when he says that autoethnography "is not always about finding solutions, sometimes it is to make you aware of the uncertainty." He also thinks that the object of the autoethnographic research should be "something we have been through, something that is behind." Back then, I needed a new way to process the whole experience, and a writing project helped me to conduct my internal research.

3   A MAP is Always a Treasure

I am sitting on this airplane because I am ready to face waves and storms, and I believe I am taking all precautions not to get overwhelmed. Luckily it is just an internal debate; since we are traveling over the Atlantic Ocean maybe it would not be the most popular metaphor to share openly.

Speaking of the ocean, when I think of myself as part of an emergency response, the furthest from my mind is the rescuer that jumps in the water with a lifesaver from an airplane or a helicopter. I see myself more like arriving at a harbor and getting into a vessel to navigate the waves to reach the spot. Then I envision myself cooperating with a local crew, maybe with different views but rooted in the culture, who know the coast, the particular weather conditions and the local rules of navigation. I won't be the lone rescuer. There cannot be lone rescuers in this field. I think I can be a legitimate member of the crew of this vessel though, because I believe myself to be an experienced sailor and I bring a MAP with me. What a pleasure to recognize the Lion speaking here, answering the important question: "Will your work be added value?" Then, the Scarecrow could take over by checking the prerequisite list that a professional should consider prior any crisis intervention (VanFleet and Mochi, 2014, p.174):

- proper training *checked*,
- relevant experience *checked*,
- being grounded locally *checked*,

- working within a structure that can ensure duration and perspective *checked*.

I see the screen in front of me with its high-tech map, and I think my personal added value is the MAP I take with me. It is the result of My Awareness Process and it is not at all as fancy and detailed as that one. My MAP is more like a collection of reference points, like the constellations for sailors. My therapist refers to it as a flexible map, like the one Columbus used. He probably built his assumptions on different information and reasoning, maybe he also had some written documents to hand, but definitely not a proper map. He took enormous risks during his journey, and I think that my first task as a member of the crew is working to minimize such risks as much as possible. *Looking for reference points and elaborating a conceptual MAP of intervention together*, this can be a good starting point in the work with my new colleagues tomorrow.

Some years ago, Isabella Cassina and I combined our experiences and elaborated a model of intervention. It includes a suggestion of principles, activities and techniques suitable for different phases. It is as dynamic and consistent ensemble of elements that help to orient the crew as the constellations are for sailors. It is not a precise plan to implement, nor a defined project one can use in every circumstance and country. It is not a detailed travel book. No one can predict and dictate every single step that has to be taken. It is a MAP you are completing as you go, like the old ones you can see in museums.

Our role as trainers in a crisis setting is to have and provide reference points that are as clear as possible. Like road signs, they should offer rapid comprehension to ensure safety and promote orientation. I have seen exceptions though: "Monday to Friday you can turn right with the exception of Thursday at 5pm and..." In some cases, there is no way you can drive and understand instantly what you are supposed to do. The same goes for navigation. At this point, someone could argue: "Do not take any new route if you don't have a map or without knowing how to read the one you have!" And my comment would be: "This is exactly why you need experienced sailors to help building orientation skills and to give support in confusing or dangerous moments." In my future Manual for Crisis Interventions, I will dedicate a chapter to this topic.

Virgil wrote: "Fortunate is the man who can understand the cause of things" (cited in Drewes and Schaefer, 2014), and I will add: "Lucky also those who are skilled in summarizing and clarifying their concepts!" I recently realized how much it took me to get my reference points this clear. If I read my old reports, I see that so many elements I teach and use now in training and projects were already "between the lines" a long time ago. The difference is that now everything is more organized and evident for me to use and address.

In all my work in crisis situations, I have always inserted a strong capacity-building component, but looking back, I realize the trainings I presented were not always complete. Practice in the field, compared to the theoretical component, was always richer, with a lot of practical examples, modeling, reinforcing that was not explicitly addressed and underlined in the training room. I could demonstrate more than I could explain. The project I developed had always clear phases with related specific actions and a vision of the entire process. I had the knowledge to explain, support, discuss each step, but I was missing the lucid and immediate concepts to refer to.

On the one hand, I could easily translate the different phases of the project and the overall process into action, on the other I could not present them as accurately from a theoretical point of view. There was a tangible practical content, but the "abstract" was "absent:" the ability to go straight to the point and describe long and complex research with just few lines. It was more like an articulated story without a particular and lucid moral, exactly like the complicated road signs we sometimes encounter, the ones you need more time to understand and which make your journey longer. Maybe I was not very skilled in summarizing or I was not paying much attention to this aspect, or simply I was committed to too many things at once.

Meanwhile my neighbor reads and I sip my coffee. I actually see the crude and simple truth in front of me: I was not able to get to the point and extract the abstract of the research for two reasons. First, the work was not finished, but was under construction. If I think of my working experience as a story, I can say that every new work, colleague and challenge added new pieces to the script and it took time to collect the narrative for the different paragraphs. Second, the actual work on the story and the research component were missing. The different lines of the story were not combined and, like a treasure, the essence of the story was yet to be found. Only after you have assembled all your data and completed your research you can write a comprehensive and meaningful abstract. The truth is that the elements of the story for me remained mostly implicit, preserved in some part of my body and brain. I missed the process that helps to make the implicit become explicit, which rewards you with emotional awareness and learning experiences.

Not exactly, but project after project, my line was something like: "We got there, good. It was hard but we made it." In practical terms the case was closed, then the usual self-care maintenance, and I moved onto another commitment. For a long time, I did not make space to reflect on the experiences. I missed the occasion, or maybe the nerve, to sit and think about what had helped us. What significant elements guided us there? What can be useful in other situations? I did not make the mistake of thinking that this is the kind of work you can copy and paste, but also I did not research deeper and review the experience and learn more for it. I did not work to create the My Awareness Process. It was like being in the flow and navigating the moment with the support of explicit knowledge and several implicit references and principles.

"Easy writing leads to hard reading. Hard writing leads to easy and more accessible reading" (Billig, 2010, cited in Bochner, 2016). The hard and regular processing was missing. Somehow I skipped the deep, hard work that brings lucidity. With time it came along, piece after piece, working with Isabella, supervisors and therapists. It was not really sought after, but happened mostly by wandering and digging here and there. One day, when I will have more time, I want to write something brief about the difference between Tourists, Wanderers and Researchers. I think it is a tripartition that can be applied in different fields, and I can learn a lot from it.

4   When Falling in Love is Not Convenient

Maybe because I like sailing or because the view of the sea from my window inspires me, this navigating metaphor sticks in my head. It is fascinating how every single action and little part of the boat has a name, even the apparently most insignificant piece of rope. This is to reduce confusion and mistakes that might obstruct navigation and create risks for the passengers and the vessel. Indeed, in crisis work, our actions can have a profound impact for good or bad. This implies a lot of responsibility and, as such, it requires the ability to respond. If we are not aware of what we are doing and we do not have references, we do not just risk failure, but could cause serious damage. I think of the Inter-Agency Standing Committee's guidelines (2007, p.2), which list "humanitarian aid-induced social problems" as the categories of problems following a disaster. The Inter-Agency Standing Committee, as many Health institutions, states the principle *primum non nocere*: "first do not harm."

The primary objective of any intervention is to prevent additional stress and damage. In fancy terms, we can say that the intervention should be part of the solution and not part of the problem. In our training for professionals, when we present the background of a crisis scenario, we underline how bureaucracy, lack of community involvement and other factors can create unintentional harm to survivors. We name one of the specific risks "falling in love with our tools" (Mochi and Cassina, 2018). This alludes to the proclivity to like a protocol or a technique so much that one applies it everywhere, without considering the objective circumstances of the context: "This is what I know, what I like, and I want to apply it."

The means to a goal becomes the goal itself. Paraphrasing Maslow, it is because one has a hammer and *wants* to use it[7].

I have witnessed many times how the wish to help, the love for our tools or confusing the maps with the territory[8] can worsen risky situations for both survivors and helpers. Every time I touch this point, it opens an effusion of bitterness in me. This is the only part of this work I do not appreciate. So many episodes that made me quite angry run through my thoughts. The worst is when ineffective, risky and damaging interventions are even promoted as successful. At times, it seems it does not count what you do or what results you get, but what you say you did and how loudly you say it. My therapist almost a decade ago said to me: "You cannot change certain dynamics, what you can do is to write something about them. That won't change the facts, but at least you will be able to say, I told you so!"

Sitting here, looking out the window, I can hear another part of me saying, "Claudio, who are you to judge? You are not supposed to state what is good or not." Moreover, Isabella and I developed a model of intervention. We consider it flexible, amendable. However, still there are phases, tools to consider in different moments. Are we secretly in love with it? Are we like those I criticize? Do I think we are the "good" ones? The silence of the situation makes this questions echo in my head. I can imagine the debate in the Land of Oz:

Scarecrow: "Alert here. Alarm rigidity. This guy became quite presumptuous."

Tin Man: "Come on, he is just frustrated. He has been in so many situations he could not control."

Lion: "He is just stating his points. He has gained a lot of experience, after all."

---

[7] The text refers to Abraham Maslow quote: "I suppose it is tempting, if the only tool you have is a hammer, to treat everything as if it were a nail" (1966, p.16).

[8] "The map is not the territory" was coined by the scientist Alfred Korzybski in 1933. It is also one of the founding principles of Neuro-linguistic Programming. It underlines the "difference between our experience of the world, and the world itself" (Dilts 1994, p.153).

Toto: "Guys, you are taking it all too seriously. What's wrong with playing with ideas? Give him time so he can clarify his thoughts."

Thanks Toto, we should never take ourselves too seriously. I agree with Perry (2020), who said, "All models are wrong, but some are useful." Models or references are not the reality, as a map is not the territory, but they help us to move in difficult circumstances and unknown spaces. This is especially so in crisis situations in which every circumstance is different. You can be a sailor or a skipper, but there are different seas with different coastlines, rocks, reefs, and regular or sudden changes in currents and weather conditions. Crisis interventions cannot be confined into one single method or approach, but I am still convinced that certain elements should be present. I am a Play Therapist and I believe in the *Therapeutic Powers of Play* (Schaefer, 1993; Schaefer and Drewes, 2014). In different ways and stages, playing can support children and adults during and after a crisis. Nevertheless, I do not think this approach can be applied in every phase of the intervention in a pre-established way.

A few days after the earthquake that struck the historic city of Bam in Iran, I remember a guy from a big news agency approaching me in the midst of a camp: "Are you working in the psychosocial field? When did you arrive? Do you work with children?" The summary of his talk was, they wanted to see children playing because they needed images of resilient children. That day, I spent my entire time in the camp surrounded by rubble. I met first one family and, after a delicious tea and a long conversation, they introduced me to the camp leader and then to a sort of a committee. Between one meeting and the other, some children invited the translator and me to play soccer. I think after several hours in the camp, parents and children started to get used to us.

We were planning to involve the people from that camp in a project and, at some point, also to organize play activities. We had boxes of toys ready, but it was not yet the moment to bring them with me; I was resolved not to play with children unless invited.

Also, back then play was one of my favorite working tools, but I was aware we were entering people's life spaces after a disaster that had resulted in thousands of deaths, and devastated most of the city.

Our plan was to introduce ourselves and show respect for the condition of individuals and for their culture. We tried to become more familiar and predictable for the survivors and, at the same time, we wanted to understand more about the overall situation. I believe this approach did not cause any damage or misunderstanding, but on the contrary brought a lot of learning and set a good foundation for the future steps of our project. At the time, and now, the idea is to be supportive not by instigating a single game in order to provide some kind of immediate relief, but, both practically and metaphorically, by organizing tournaments, in order to build play sanctuaries and a culture of play that would remain long after our departure.

At some point during the training I think I might use this anecdote as an example. It may be a good way to underline that there are many different ways to intervene in crisis, but at the foundation there should be some key components:

- respect for the individual conditions and culture,

- understanding the complexity of needs in order to be effective, and

- safety for survivors and for the professionals involved.

This is clear. What is not yet clear is, if after twenty years of work in the field, have I become more aware of my beliefs, or if I am just more rigid and I see what I want to see? I guess the first hypothesis is the right one and I could prove I am not in love with my own views by researching more on the topic. This time the perspective of "the big trauma experts" cannot help. This is something domestic, personal. I guess I have to start from an internal kind of research. If it is true that "we grasp our lives in a narrative" (Taylor, cited in Bochner and Riggs, 2014, p.195), then I should commit to writing something. Professional writing has helped me in the past. Taylor says, "In order to have a sense of who we are, we have to have a notion of how we have become, and of where we are going" (Ibid).

How tempting it is to write now about examples of dangerous or inconsistent practices but I do not want to take time to underline others' wrongdoings. It would be like digging a mine with the intent to proving there is nothing to find there. Not a smart move. Following Taylor's words, I am going to start my own research, detecting my own mistakes.

There is so much in writing and I am going to use it as an inquiry tool. The entire preparation process that leads to writing, the research into the experiences, the internal debate, the studies are all great ways to examine and understand and, as Chang (2007) wrote, "self-reflection and self-examination are the keys to self-understanding" (p.52). This is, in part, what I am doing now. Also, sharing the work once completed, with the possibility to have comments and feedback, is good material for my understanding. I like the perspective on writing that Bochner and Ellis (ICQM, 2014) have: "To open up a conversation, stimulate the reader to relate." Actually, this is exactly the same view I have for the training process I am going to present in a few days. Share reference points to open a discussion and set the base to co-construct a path, to open up new possibilities. Writing down my notes, examples, and relevant theories and put it all together as if I am writing a book is a fantastic way for me to clarify my point of view and to state my uncertainties. And then who knows. Let me read that piece from Bochner, as I think it is so appropriate and meaningful for me now:

> Moments before he died, Tolstoy remarked, "I don't know what I'm supposed to do." Human beings are born not knowing and we still don't know when we die. But, between birth and death we have to choose something to do. I chose the human sciences because I thought they could show me life as it really is. But I found out I wanted to do something more than merely receive this knowledge; I wanted to react to it, converse with it, and apply it. But the ruling paradigm encouraged replication, not conversation. Now I know what

I want to do is make people feel stuff, continue my quest to put into circulation self-clarifying and transforming stories, and keep alive the conversation in the human sciences about what can make life good. That may not be what I am supposed to do, but it does feel like the right thing to do (Bochner, 2016, p.305).

5   Three Dimensions of a Good Practice

I am getting closer to my destination. Where are we going to start, and which direction will we take? I had asked myself these questions several other times, especially where the disaster was really massive and the expectation from my employer unrealistic. Port-au-Prince, a few days after the earthquake, comes to my mind. The moment arrived in Haiti and stepped out of the airport the scenario was terrible, with thousands of tents and millions of needs everywhere. My thought was exactly the same as I have now: "Where do we start?" Through the experience and countless moments of doubt, I reached the conviction that a valid starting point is embracing and applying the core elements of a good practice and only later along the way focus on those considered to be best practices.

In the greatest moment of uncertainty, stick to the principles. I will start the training by exploring participants' ideas of good practice, with some activities and sharing my own perspective on its basic elements. I will support my point of view with personal experiences in the field, theoretical and scientific notions. To make my work easier, I will write down the narratives (in italics in the present text) for the examples and also the comments I want to be sure to make. I could also write down the slides (in gray boxes) with the concepts I want to share. This preparation is a total novelty for me, so here we go, a new story is starting: *good practice involves three dimensions: respect, effectiveness and safety.*

5.1 Respect

I think of when I'd arrived soon after the earthquake in Bam, Iran. Apart from the mosque, all the city was destroyed and almost half of the population died. In my first project there, I was required to collect information and provide initial psychological support. I carried with me my "working bag" with different trauma and post-disaster psychological tools, but confronted with the vastness of pain and basic needs, it just did not feel right to undertake interviews, collect data or apply any kind of protocol or procedure. I had my evidence-based material with me but I left it in my tent. Was I uncertain or inexperienced in the face of such magnitude of human suffering? Did I have the need to understand because I was overwhelmed or confused by the destruction? My idea, many years later, is that I have just been respectful.

The word "respect" has such a fascinating etymology. It originates from the Latin *re-spicere*, "to look back." In front of a person or a situation, instead of proceeding forward, we stop to give proper attention because the person has special worth or interest for us. We pause in order to adjust our attitude or behavior. Respect implies the need to take a moment to reflect, research and evaluate doubts in order to apply what is considerate and courteous according to the situation, the individual conditions, the person's culture and uniqueness. To introduce this point to my colleagues, I think I might share an example.

A few days after a terrible earthquake, I was in the field doing my assessment, meeting people in their place of living. I remember, in the evening, the rescuers were throwing blankets to the survivors from their trucks without stopping. Several survivors were upset because it was getting cold and they did not have anything to cover themselves. I recall in particular an old lady telling me that she tried to reach the truck to get a blanket but she was too slow to either follow it or to grasp one of the blankets lying on the ground.

The needs were huge and the emergency team had the best intentions to provide as many blankets in the shortest possible time. Still, for the old lady, the result of this action was that she felt humiliated, more helpless, despairing, stressed and colder than before. If the rescuers had taken the time "to look back," they could easily have realized that part of their action, at least, was fruitless.

Being prompt and responsive to the needs is important in an emergency, but psychosocial interventions require respect prior to any other practice. To summarize some of the points we have been discussing, let's consider the following definition of respect taken from the American Psychological Association Dictionary (2020):

"Attitude of, or behavior demonstrating, esteem, honor, regard, concern, and other such positive qualities toward an individual or entity. Respect can serve an important purpose in interpersonal and intergroup relations by aiding in communication, for example. According to many theorists and practitioners, it is considered to play a crucial role as a bidirectional process in psychotherapy."

5.2 Effectiveness

A good practice should be effective in reaching its predefined objectives.

> "Efficacy defines the adequacy of the results obtained in reaching the specific and pre-planned objectives" (Naiaretti, Sagramoso and Solaro del Borgo, 2006, p.99).

We know so much about effective and evidence based practices; there is a lot of research available on different categories of problems.

Efficacy relies on a vast repertoire of skills, but it is just one component of effectiveness.

In general, if you have to play a soccer match, it can be good to count on Ronaldo or Messi[9] on your team, but they are less useful or relevant if you are going to play rugby.

An intervention is likely to be effective only if it addresses needs that are relevant for its intended recipients.

> "Relevance defines the adequacy of the intervention/project and its results in solving the identified problems" (Ibid).

---

[9] Ronaldo and Messi are popular football players; they are considered by many the best in their generation.

An intervention can be relevant if needs are assessed carefully. Especially in a crisis situation, we might think it is possible and maybe easy to anticipate which needs are sensitive, but actually our work is about understanding and not assuming.

I think I wrote something similar with Risë several years ago. Let me check to include it in my presentation:

> "Interventions start with the needs of the survivors. It is tempting to assume that as mental health professionals we know what is needed in post-disaster situations. Because every disaster and every survivor is unique, this assumption must be avoided" (Mochi and VanFleet, 2009, p.17).

I believe I understood this point well in my first international work as coordinator. It was in the former Yugoslavia after the Balkan War in the 1990s. I was around thirty and didn't have any sensational prior experience in this field. This example might open interesting discussions.

It was in Europe, several years after a war. The association that hired me had worked for years in the area to support refugees and Internally Displaced People to adapt to the situation and improve their condition. Different programs were implemented, such as micro projects, financed relocation outside the collective centers[10], provision of working tools and construction material, and delivery of other goods. It was a considerate plan that worked in consultation with some of the beneficiaries. For the rest of the people, the support brought some relief but only as long as the assistance was provided.

It was the beginning of 2000 and psychosocial interventions were not consolidated practices, but their team started to think that the psychological component played an important role there. One short psychological intervention was tried and, after that, it was decided to initiate a psychosocial assessment and a related project. I arrived

---

[10] "Collective centers are defined as pre-existing buildings and structures used for the collective and communal settlement of a displaced population in the event of a conflict or natural disaster" (United Nations High Commissioner for Refugees, 2015).

without a ready-made recipe. They put no pressure on me and I took time to understand the context and the beneficiaries' condition, their strength and mindset.

A lot of time was also dedicated to building a common mutual enriching perspective with the team, but writing about this now would distract from the point.

The people living in the collective centers had very hard and even horrific past experiences and, in addition to that, all of them were experiencing burdensome, everyday struggles. Whatever was going on in their present did not help to get relief from the past and, on the contrary, made their life even more difficult.

It took us almost three months to meet all the families more than once. Did it take so long because as coordinator I was not that experienced? This happened almost two decades ago; with the experience and learning I gained, would it be faster now?

We spent three months with regular fieldwork aimed at knowing each other, building trust, engaging them, providing initial psychological support, and collecting information about their assets, needs, perspectives and mindset.

During the assessment, the actual psychosocial support project had already started, and at the same time we were building our in-house capacities and setting the base for the development of phases and local assets. Now that I think about this, I realize that process was the first rough version of the approach "Coping with the present while building for the future" (CPBF) (Mochi and Cassina, 2018).

Among the many relevant pieces of information, what they disclosed about their future perspectives was very significant. The vast majority among the hundreds of adults involved expressed a profound sense of helplessness. They had reached a point where they believed that there was nothing they could do to improve their circumstances, and it was meaningless to try any longer. They had completely lost hope (VanFleet and Mochi, 2015, p.170). There was not the idea that in the future the situation could improve or there was no future perspective at all. There was also a general feeling of distrust toward the Government and the Humanitarian associations.

"Chronic and unpredictable stress may be more likely to create a series of enduring personality changes and disrupt the individual's basic sense of trust in relationship and confidence in the future" (McFarlane and De Girolamo, 2007, p.138). Their traumatic experiences, and everything that followed them, had imposed a high cost also on their mindset that revealed signs of alteration in the sense of self (helplessness and ineffectiveness), in the perception of others (lack of trust) and in the system of values (foreshortened future, loss of previous beliefs) (van der Kolk, 2000, p.10, and 2002, pp.139-40).

The previous programs, focused on assisting and providing external solutions, didn't change their attitude toward life and maybe even reinforced their helplessness and state of dependency. The provision of financial and material support, occupation, home and working tools was meeting certain needs but was neglecting others, in particular their need to regain a sense of being active, capable and effective. They had the necessity to focus on the present, to believe they could make some changes in their life. They had to recover a future perspective, and ownership in the solutions.

At this point of the training, I can include the presentation with a reference from the Inter-Agency Standing Committee about the importance of active participation in any psychosocial projects:

"Participation should enable different sub-groups of local people to retain or resume control over decisions that affect their lives, and to build the sense of local ownership that is important for achieving program quality, equity and sustainability" (Inter-Agency Standing Committee, 2007, p. 11).

The final project took account of the needs we found and, even if it wasn't well funded, it was quite articulated including basic material support together with a psychological component. There were many initiatives with family projects, group activities for children and adults.

Here it would be just perfect to start talking about "sustainability" and "capacity building," but I guess it might be confusing.

We had a saying back then that can summarize the essence of the program: "No psychological intervention can be effective if your window glass is broken and outside is freezing!" Now I can also add there was no space for improvement by just fixing the glass and providing a heater. Effectiveness is a necessary component of a good practice, and it can be defined as the realization of objectives relevant to the beneficiaries of the intervention. It relies on the ability to carefully assess the needs and to plan and implement a suitable course of action.

I believe the implicit components of this concept are flexibility, capability to adjust, and a solid and updated repertoire of skills to be used consistently with local needs. A fixed pre-planned program will never work in-depth. It would be a weak foundation for any process and not completely a respectful practice. I have so many practical examples to add... I remember when I was... Fine, the Scarecrow just reminded me to focus on the memories that are useful for my work here!

5.3 Safety

As humans we are able to function properly only in certain conditions. And one of them is when we are in a condition of safety. We can learn, explore, connect with others, regulate our emotions, soothe ourselves, access our resources only when we feel safe. As Stephen Porges (2011, p. 20) clearly describes with his Polyvagal theory: "We are genetically wired to detect safety, danger, or threat, even below the level of consciousness." This process that continuously appraises the risks is called Neuroception. Taking on Porges' work, we can use his metaphor of the Traffic Light (Porges, cited in Kestly, 2014, p. 17).

Our preferred way of functioning is safety. In that moment our Social Engagement System (SES) is active and, like when we are in a junction with a green light, we are free to proceed and decide where to go and what to do. On the contrary, when we perceive a danger, we activate another branch of our nervous system (the sympathetic accelerator). In that moment, our mobilization response is online and we become:

> "Hyper-vigilant—yellow light—with increased body sensations, emotional reactivity, intrusive images, and cognitive impairment" (Kestly 2016, p. 20).

If this way of reacting fails, if our fight or flee response does not work to make us feel safer, we automatically move to the third option, the parasympathetic brake with fear of death, which brings us a shutdown state:

> "Immobilization—red light—with decreased or even eliminated sensation, incapacitated cognitive processing, reduced physical movement, a sense of emptiness or deadness, passivity, and numbing of emotions" (Ibid).

When using the term "safety," we are not talking just of the physical component, but also include the psychological one. Our perception of safety goes beyond our field of awareness.

My mind goes to those kids frozen in the school class in Nigeria where their teachers where shouting and threatening them with a long bamboo stick to have their attention. I think as well of the situations where kids were humiliated just to make a point. Not a tangible threat there, but most of them felt so scared that they had zero chance to actively participate, learn and thrive properly. All they cared about was trying to protect themselves and finishing the class as soon as possible. There are a number of other examples I could relate here but I have to be careful in choosing. I do not want to touch something too sensitive too soon. Anyway, I think that the need of psychological safety for children at this point will be quite clear and we could start reflecting on how to provide it.

The first time I was confronted with such a dilemma, I was working in Palestine in the midst of ongoing conflict. In natural disasters, one of the priorities of the intervention is to create a safe space. But what can we do when nobody can ensure physical safety? After a long process, the viable solution I found at the time was relying on the powers of play and the power of relationships (Mochi, 2009). Many years later, I am even more convinced of this.

I would like to share an experience I had found very insightful. It was in a conflict zone where we worked to develop psychosocial centers for children. Children's lives were affected by a variety of limitations, and in addition there were frequent military operations in the area that represented actual danger to them and local workers. The situation was very sensitive, but during playtime, children looked joyfully engaged in their activities. It seemed they could overcome the limitations and the fears of daily life. They were playing, for instance, the role of powerful and strong characters, winning battles, creating fantastic scenarios where life could offer plenty of positive opportunities. During the next several days, we will talk in more detail about the powers of play, but for the moment I would like to share an episode that really impressed me.

During one of these playtimes, we heard a loud explosion. All of the children stopped playing at once, and I stopped too. I was sitting on the ground and, as far as I remember, the children all looked suddenly at my colleague M. I still have goosebumps when I revisit the scene in my mind. M. did not blink, he did not appear nervous or worried, and continued with the activity he had been engaged in. After a few moments, all the children resumed their play. I did not know back then of Porges and the Polyvagal theory, but it was so clear for me that as referent adults, our relationship is a safety bank for children. The moment children saw M. calm and at ease, they realized the place was safe for them; they got the "green light" to resume their play.

As humans, we have the incredible gift of being able to influence the green light for others. According to Porges (2011, p. 93), we can use direct modalities like play to provide safety, or indirect or passive modalities that develop through the relationship we establish. Once we neuroperceive safety and our SES is active, we can promote its activation in other people.

The combination of our posture, gestures, the tone of our voice, our facial expressions, the way we use proximity can have to potential to increase the neuroception of safety in others, or exactly the opposite. We are going to work and share ideas on both active and passive ways to recruit SES in others. This topic will accompany each and every aspect of our project. For the moment, I would like you to think of the importance of our own psychological safe place. It is only when we are able to activate our own SES and send clues of safety that we can support our clients. We will talk soon also about self-care, but first let me add another little piece of experience.

My colleague M. was living in a very difficult situation. The location where he lived was not immune to the harshness of the conflict, but nevertheless it was peaceful, comfortable and well taken care of. He had a rich network of family and friends all around. I had the impression that he carefully created his own safe psychological place. I do not know how natural or how much effort was put into that, but it seemed to me that he and his family were managing their location and lifestyle to fill it with a positive and regenerating atmosphere. They controlled and managed what they could.

In few days, you will meet Isabella. One of the things I am learning from her is to be proactive in creating a context where we can feel better, be calmer and more productive. She does not suffer from the context, simply because she does her best to change what she can. And guess what? As Robert Brooks (2015, p. 10) said, resilient people spend energy in controlling what they can. People less resilient do just the opposite. Creating our own safe place is a long but necessary work. Many aspects can contribute, or be detrimental, starting from the physical location.

How little I knew at that time about how to create a safe place! Even now, I am passive and automatic in certain aspects of my life. "Take your stance, where is your ground? Remember: your safety is in your position, you can be safe only when you are well balanced and grounded on your feet!" I am a hopeless amateur boxer but I got several pieces of wisdom from my coach. Feeling grounded and stable is essential. In crisis work, it means to be part of a structure rooted in a culture, to have clarity about the terms of our role, of what is required and what we can *actually* do.

Before doing an activity, let's emphasize a couple of points: the powers of play can be unlocked when we feel safe, but specific play activities help us to feel safer. There is no place that is safe once and for all. It is not about reaching a safe mountain or an island. It is more like navigating, adjusting to the territory, the streams and the weather conditions. We do our best to be as in control of the vessel as possible, while going everywhere we want. There are peaceful waters, but no water is immune to threat. Safety as life (let me remove the word "life" from my note, since I do not want to play guru) requires continuous adjustments, and so effort and attention. This is why we need to work in extending our experience and ability in developing occasions to promote safety in others and in ourselves.

We build our safe place moment by moment, and all of us has an individual way to obtain, maintain and regain our own safety. I would like to share one more possibility for developing this sense of safety. I am going to read a story titled The Magic Home: A Displaced Boy Finds a Way to Feel Better[11] (Cassina, 2020a) and then invite you to do an activity along with that.

5.4 Relationship

"The best predictor of how you're doing in the present isn't your history of adversity, it's your history of connectedness," Perry (2020) says, and this makes a lot of sense. I think I have to add an element here, because all dimensions of good practice take place on a common ground: the relationship. At the same time, their inter-relation nourishes certain qualities i that are essential in any therapeutic process. Our nature moves us and forces us to rely on others for support and safety, and allows us access to our resources

---

[11] *The Magic Home* (Cassina, 2020a) is an illustrated psychoeducational book for children that suggests a very interesting closing activity. I am not going to add any detail about it because this would be revealing the end of the story. Nevertheless, I decided to mention it because this core activity is deeply related to the concept of psychological safety and the importance of the relationship. Most likely, it is something I would suggest at this stage of the training.

and capabilities. Our health and recovery from hurdles is based on positive relationships. How all dimensions interact with one another is so beautifully clear in my head. How to convey this to my new colleagues, though? It would be fantastic to quote Allen or Rogers about the importance of the relationship and to move on. Maybe it would be better to share some ideas and work on them to define a common foundation. Let me write down an anecdote that might make sense. I am afraid I will be nick-named "Homer" after all these stories!

I was working in a fairly conservative Islamic area. The location was remote and, according to the information I received, the local community was quite reluctant to interact with foreigners. My task was to establish psychosocial centers in different villages. I had a timeline, an assessment to write, several trainings to present, and activities to plan. My starting point was selecting a village and introducing myself to the village leader and, after several meetings, asking to meet the local teachers. Following the local cultural practice, we set up a formal meeting in the space of the mosque. Instead of four people, all the women of the village came. We spent the entire day talking. I had the idea of speaking about the project, focusing on adult and child traumatic reactions; yet, as I recall, I put aside all the notes, scripts and information I had intended to gather in order to follow the group's interests. We were "simply" getting to know each other. I was aware I could not start the project using any of the ways I had used in other countries; it had to be their way. The time taken to understand and follow the local culture was the key to setting up the foundation for the entire project. The regular meetings with the chief gave me access to the big group, the big group to the smaller groups and the families and, once I had met the whole community, we started working together. This in turn opened the way for me to the next villages.

Nothing was preplanned in this process, or, to be honest, all the planning was changed because it would have never been applicable. And still we progressed in a way that satisfied everybody. All pieces of the process were grounded in the relationship, and everything we did or did not do had the scope to make it more trustful. Respect, effectiveness[12] *and safety made that possible.*

At this point, even if I am aware that the power of relationship can only be deeply understood through personal experience, and by paying attention to our Company of Oz, I would like to add a theoretical framework to our conversation. It is fundamental to underline that one of the most important aspects of our work is to emphasize the relationships we build. All support to the beneficiaries is conveyed through the interactions positive relationships make possible. I will start with a philosophical quote:

"Everything can be found in isolation except sanity" (Friedrich Nietzsche, cited in Cozolino, 2016, p. 13).

I will then add citations from different authors to underline that the need for others, to feel safe and protected, to learn and to recover from our problem is not just theoretical but actually deeply rooted in our genes.

We are social beings. Our learning and the possibility we have to adapt to different situations happens through relationships. In fact, the brain is defined as "a social organ of adaptation, shaped by evolution to connect with and change through interactions with others" (Ibid).

Our brains have the ability "to attune and learn from one another in the service of adaptive change" (Ludy-Dobson and Perry 2010, p. 26). It is our social nature that makes us a very distinctive species. Ludy-Dobson and Perry maintain that "the most important property of humankind is the capacity to form and maintain relationships. These relationships are absolutely necessary for any of us to survive" and feel safe. In fact, "healthy relational interactions are our protective factors" that help us to regain a neuroception of safety and "thrive following trauma and loss." We are wired to respond positively to other humans even in very difficult circum-stances. It is important for us to consider that research shows:

---

[12] Here "effectiveness" is meant as the realization of relevant objectives, and it is based on the ability to carefully assess the community's needs, and accordingly to plan and implement a suitable course of action.

"The presence of familiar people projecting the social-emotional cues of acceptance, understanding, compassion, and empathy calm the stress response of the individual" (Ludy-Dobson and Perry, 2010, pp. 26-7).

Change and resilience, and so the effectiveness of an intervention, are built and achieved through connections. All studies on resilience show that the ability to deal with and overcome difficult circumstances is based on the possibility of connecting with at least one caring, reliable and predictable person (Brooks, 2015; Perry, 2020).

"Safe and attuned connections create the possibility for both short-term and long-lasting modification of the brain. Through the security of a safe relationship, something new can be introduced into a previously closed and dysfunctional system" (Cozolino, 2016, p. 15).

For these reasons, every interaction should be seen as an opportunity to reinforce the beneficiaries of our project, and make them feel accepted, cared for, respected, safe, understood and positively regarded (Brooks, 2015, p. 11).

To conclude and summarize, healthy and supportive relationships are necessary elements to set in motion a process of successful adaptation, whether they come from the immediate or the extended support system. This process can obviously be articulated and developed in different ways, for instance applying various techniques and approaches. Nevertheless, I believe the foundation on which this process is built is more solid if every step is grounded in respect, effectiveness and safety. The "ordinary magic" can take place along this way.

"Resilience does not come from rare and special qualities, but from the everyday magic of ordinary, normative human resources in the minds, brains and bodies of children, in their families, and in their communities" (Masten, 2001, p. 235).

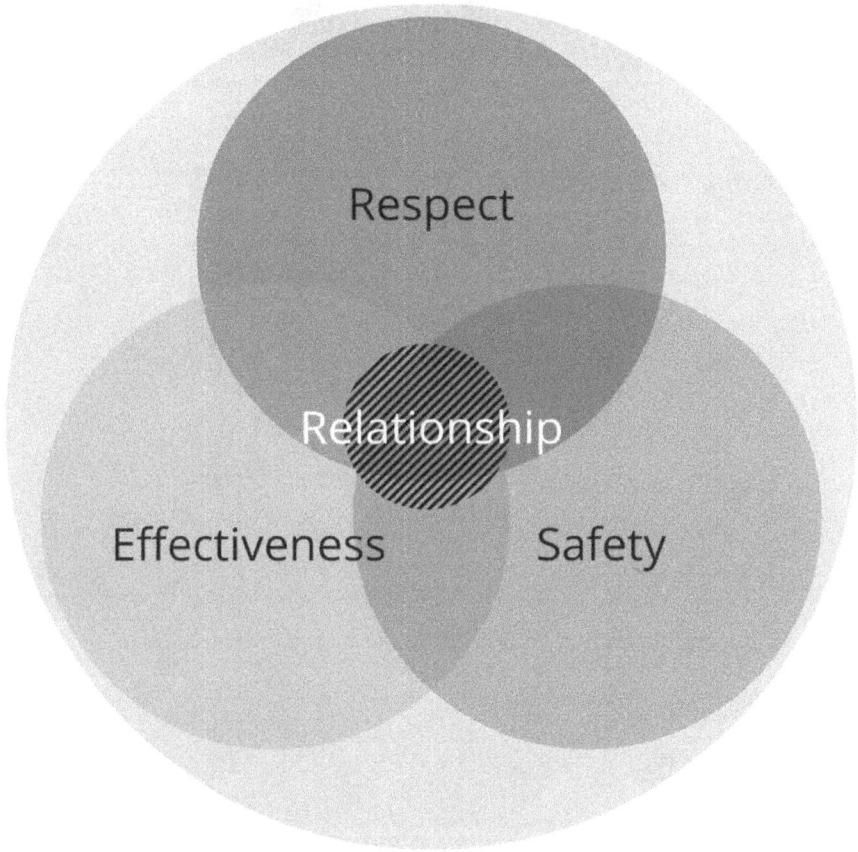

Fig. 1: Three dimensions of a good practice.

6 Coping with the Present While Building for the Future

I can see the islands; I understand we are not too far off now. I think that on this plane trip, I set a good base for our work, especially from the mental point of view. Being more prepared, I will have more energy and focus to dedicate to the work. I will just write down the list of the specific reference points to consider in crisis:

- needs assessment
- community mobilization
- capacity building
- play
- Play Therapy and Expressive Arts Therapy
- uninterrupted monitoring
- self-care

Maybe I have the time to work on two of them before landing. I will choose play and self-care. I think an introduction is necessary. I have to present the wider approach that connects all the other points: Coping with the present while building for the future (CPBF) (Mochi and Cassina, 2018). It is like our mantra in this field of work (Cassina, 2020b, p. 6).

The Theater Metaphor

I imagine crisis intervention as a co-construction of a stage upon which to narrate and produce different plays. The first moment is dedicated to preparing the base for the stage, involving actors and scriptwriters. Then it is necessary to get all permissions to present the play, involve other people to act, support and follow it. When all is as ready as possible, make the last arrangements to the stage and perform the first act. The first act is a source of inspiration for the second. New lines and plots develop from the actors and the audience during the play itself. What happens in the performance influences the next scenography, script, and all stage arrangements. It is a very creative, but also organized process. The first act of the play is also dedicated to determining what is going to happen in the second act, or to decide if indeed there should be a further act. Once the first performance is finished, it is already time to decide what will happen the next day and, if required, to make the last adaptations to the scene, edit the script, and rehearse. Every day you play and pick up all sensitive information while building the base for the next act. In this way, the play is always responsive and engaging.

The whole play is not pure improvisation, because there are always specific themes in the setting that evolve over time as the story develops. There are also different actors with specific talents that make the play unique. This is a specific sector of acting where the aim is the involvement of the audience more than their entertainment and, of course, the play is real life rather than fiction. To be a good performer in these scenarios, you need a combination of adaptability and preparation.

I am glad I recalled this metaphor I have used at other times (Mochi and Cassina, 2018) and it makes total sense to me. It fits with the nature of crisis work, which requires multi-layered interventions and parallel processes. It is also compatible with the idea that when working through human relationships, we need to be gradual and apply all dimensions of good practice.

Through experience, we have come to perceive the intervention as a co-created developing story that cannot be rushed. I believe you can rush or accelerate only what you know. You can be faster in performing a skill if you have practiced it beforehand. You can travel briskly only if the path you choose has been defined. But this is unknown territory with no previous path, merely reference points and your preparation.

One of the most successful projects I have worked on comes to mind. My job was to plan and establish psychosocial centers in different villages. As has happened several times during various projects, we set up a center, and replicated the work in other locations. For the first center we needed quite a long time to understand the situation and the local dynamics. Slowly we started to get in contact with the community and eventually we had very good participation from different groups. The same for the second and the third village. Actually our consistency and work in the others paid off. We built some credibility and the process increased in speed.

The day of the inauguration of the fourth center, managers and supervisors came also from Europe. An interesting and dynamic celebration was organized: games, religious time, political speech, and play activities. There was a very nice atmosphere till the moment we noticed a group of bikers forming a long horizontal line approaching our fences, exactly as I have seen in the movies. Initially they just produced some noise. Suddenly, they pushed one of the fences over. With my legs almost trembling I went to put it back. Luckily none of the bikers challenged me. The atmosphere was ruined. Nobody from the authority took a position. After a few minutes, all fences were torn down and soon after we had a number of bikers riding through the tents and destroying the decorations of flowers and the art-crafts prepared by the children.

If I think of the situation, it still seems unreal to me. What did actually happen? Was it a gang? Did they want money? Were they just casual vandals? One or two days afterwards, we went to meet the group of youth and we understood that during our preparation work to open the center, we met a lot of people but we left them out. This group felt excluded and when I entered their tent I recognized one of them, for we had met before. I realized I had been superficial; I think I relied on my "automatic pilot" speeding up the process and underestimating their willingness to be part of this process. Eventually two of them became actively involved in our projects and several among the youngest participated in our activities.

There is much I could say about this process but it is necessary to focus. Let me use the remaining time to dedicated to play and self-care.

7 Three Levels of Intervention Involving Play

A range of literature and anecdotal evidence considers how and why play is important for human beings' health and development. Even if I have presented on this topic many times, I actually do not know where to begin. There are a multitude of angles to consider. Let me see what I wrote some time ago: "Play gives children the opportunity to change their passivity in the face of events into activity and creativity. In play, children can be fully themselves, elaborate and master critical events, have fun, rewrite a reality that they like better and that fits more with their feelings, aspiration and hope" (Mochi, 2009, p. 78).

I could start this part of the training with some definitions, videos, strong brain factoids, etc. Or I could just let the team experience how play activities can be powerful in relieving stress, how learning can be fun and challenges feel safe, how it is surprising and constructive to discover something new about ourselves and how play can bring individuals closer to one another.

Play is so powerful because it is part of a genetically established system common to all mammals. It is our source of joy that provides impulse to discover and connect (Panksepp and Biven, 2012).

After practice and group discussion over the various experiences, I could introduce one of my favorite definitions:

"Play is the primary way that children learn about their world, understand how things work, express themselves, develop new physical, mental and social skills and bonds" (VanFleet, 2012, p. 2).

I could then connect play to our field of work to emphasize the potential to build resilience:

Play expands the window of tolerance and allows them to exercise the vagal brake to enhance autonomic flexibility and emotional regulation.
"Through play we learn to manage pleasurable high-arousal states (sympathetic) for positive purposes and immobilization without fear for positive purpose and thus building resilience" (Kestly 2016, pp. 20-1).

At this point, I could introduce *The Therapeutic Powers of Play* (Schaefer, 1993; Schaefer and Drewes, 2014) and refer to the specific change agents in which play initiates, facilitates or strengthens their therapeutic effect.

Charles E. Schaefer and Athena A. Drewes (2014) based on the review of the literature and on their own clinical experience, identified twenty different powers that can produce change in four areas: facilitate communication, foster emotional wellness, enhance social relationships, and increase personal strengths.

I believe we are ready to consider how we can use these powers in our fieldwork. We will use play and its therapeutic powers in different phases of the crisis intervention to serve different purposes.

The Inter-Agency Standing Committee guidelines (2007, pp. 11-3) advise the application of a multi-layered approach for mental health and psychosocial support in emergencies. The guidelines suggest that all interventions should start from the provision of basic services and then move gradually toward more specialized and focused interventions. The same principle goes for the Therapeutic Powers of Play that will be applied initially to meet general and more basic needs, and shift along the process in direction of more specific needs. Figure 2 shows three possible stages of intervention:

Stage	Objectives	Activities
Initial stage Recreational activities The power of play is used for recreation, connection and assessment.	**Children:** experience a safe context, distraction, fun, release of tension, predictability, socialization with possibility to connect with peers and adults which are active in the project and the community. **Helpers:** involve children in the project. Play helps to build relationships with children and is used as initial identification of psychosocial needs.	Traditional and popular. Lighthearted, fun or sport group activities. Planned and organized by the project team or volunteers. Children can also organize them under team supervision.
Advanced stage Psychosocial activities Play based group activities to promote abilities in children and ameliorate mild psychosocial problems.	**Children:** identification and expression of emotions, self-regulation, coping skills, stress management, etc. **Helpers:** strengthen positive relationships and deeper needs assessment.	Age-specific group activities also extrapolated from different Play Therapy group activities. Each addresses a specific goal. Every session is followed by a report to document the process and results.
Specialized stage Play Therapy Different approaches to prevent or resolve psychosocial problems and psychological disorders and achieve optimal growth and development.	**Children and families:** addressing specific psychosocial needs, post-traumatic or other stress reactions, and multiple problems not improved with psychosocial activities.	Individual, group or family format using Play Therapy methodologies.

Fig. 2: The stages of a crisis intervention: focusing on the role of play.

Following an ideal process, in all three levels we should consider the approach CPBF. Each level has its specific goals and additional aims such as establishing a more solid sense of safety and trust in the relationship, and collecting more accurate information about the needs of the survivors and local partners in order to adjust the program and build capacity.

Play can have a role in regular and special circumstances by bringing joy, giving opportunity to thrive, or to relieve the most painful trauma. Nevertheless, in a crisis, play is an important reference point, but it is not a path itself. It is a component and a multifaceted tool that can be crucial in particular with children, but a project should not be an excuse to use play or apply Play Therapy. This experience showed this could be my weak point: using Play Therapy at all costs. This is why I need Toto by my side to remind me not be rigid.

A long time ago, a very large disaster hit one of the poorest countries in the world. At the time I was not aware of how much in love I was with my Play Therapy toolbox. I thought it was the ideal set of conditions to apply in a sustainable way all three levels of intervention mentioned above. I was a consultant to a big humanitarian organization and other relevant associations were considering us as a model. I thought it could be the first large intervention using Play Therapy in a sustainable way. We could train and supervise quite a number of local professionals. I was already cultivating the idea of introducing Play Therapy activities in all areas such as schools, hospitals, community centers, emergency camps, etc. I thought we could really make a difference. Theoretically, there was nothing wrong with this idea, but it was simply not possible. There were not the conditions, at least not for a year or two. Too many social needs had to be considered, the fractured social context required attention, the local partner was influential but fragile and, last but not least, my colleagues were survivors themselves with cumulative stress conditions to deal with. Everything was clearly there in front of my eyes, but it took me some time to recognize it. I was on the edge of putting pressure and imposing my ideas when luckily I stepped back.

We did not provide any specialized treatment but it was not a waste of energy. In fact, our regular play activities elevated the mood, relieved stress, and brought people closer to each other; they became more active with a renewed sense of the future. All this without stressing for more and demanding unnecessary adjustments. Reference points are important, but none of them is the actual territory. They are the means to a goal and never goals themselves. We should remember this in particular with regard to what makes us more passionate. One of my secret dreams is to make the most advanced treatments and methodologies accessible to the most remote and forgotten areas of the globe. Allow children, families and communities to reach what they could have, for instance, in the best clinics or institutions in United States or Switzerland. The idea is something like taking a piece of Switzerland somewhere else. For this reason, I need Toto and the others to look after me, because sometimes this is not possible or just not necessary.

8   *Pro per* Professional

It still comes back to me: Mr. Higgins with his passion for growing roses, practicing Tai Chi, studying, and writing his memoirs. And then Magnum fully committed in the flow of the present with his idea of writing the manual of the perfect investigator. Higgins making space for his reflecting and Magnum enjoying company, adventures, swimming. I'm growing older, and at the moment I'd rather be a combination of the two, in which proportion I would not know. Maybe 50-50 or 70-30? I feel the necessity to be in the flow, to live the entirety of the experience and I also feel a growing need to process and learn from it. It is like if you are always in the flow you might end in a place you haven't decided to be and maybe you don't even like.

I guess that, TV show aside, I have to find my own balance to suit my unique life.

Brooks states that "you can be actor of your story if you understand where you are going" (Flytenewmedia, 2020). I often have the feeling that I have been carried away and I think I should make a priority to stop regularly and think of my direction. It is decided: instead of jumping from one task to another, I am going to make space to write the manual for crisis intervention. It won't be as perfect as the one Magnum figured, but it will be at least a very good exercise for me. To keep up with the good intentions, tomorrow I am going to write a few headings... or maybe I will wait sometime since I have very long days ahead with colleagues to meet, fields to visit and a training to finalize.

In any case, today I have done a lot already. I can put my journal and my mind to rest and save myself a little. I can look if there is something new on the airplane screen. Time for relaxing, since my mind has covered "enough" ground for today. Enough? Why do I have the feeling that I am withdrawing from something interesting?

I am not tired, but I am saying to myself, "Enough for today." This is not a pause from intense reflections, it is not taking a rest, it is more a "tomorrow will do." I am merely procrastinating to avoid going further the other way. No cookies, coffee, ringing phone, blinking screens, partner around to make my escape easier. On the contrary, the restricted movements of an airplane seat are forcing me to slow down my process, and I can see what is going on. I am not in any kind of flow because instead of being focused and completely aware, I feel more like being captured by the situation and absent-mindedly carried away by a stream that will lead me to the usual tomorrow.

I have a clear picture in my mind: I am sailing peacefully on a river in my boat when I notice a very interesting tributary. I stop for a while at the bifurcation and then start navigating the new course of water, discovering a fascinating new landscape. I feel energized and happy and the more I sail the more the experience looks rich and promising. In that moment, I realize that further along, the watercourse is even more engrossing. I stop and go back to cover the usual stretch of river. I am not a fan of the extra mile to cover, but here I am giving up something promising and I know how in reality this story will continue. After the moments of profound reflection during the next few days, after work I will stay up till 1-2 am to complete the training. Old handouts will be enriched with new notes written in the long evenings. Then I will jot down endless comments on the project and about myself in my copybook with the intention of working on them once home again. Then, after returning, every excuse will be good to postpone the work and bury all the positive intentions and the documents in some drawer.

I have déjà vu: there is a younger Claudio aware of his collection of copybooks filled with illegible notes, saying during a group supervision: "I would like to improve my work by slowing down and taking time to reflect and capitalize my experience." That was no less than fifteen years ago and I was already frustrated by continually piling up experiences without the possibility of organizing and using them. I have the strong feeling that this time also, I will return with a bag filled with vibrant material to process and a genuine desire to do something different, but everything will remain unread, scattered and put aside. Ten years from now, maybe in a boat this time, I will go for a similar and interrupted journey again.

It makes no sense, does it? It is like a cook who prepares a new satisfying menu and doesn't take any notes of the process, the ingredients and the recipe. No one who wishes to be a professional would make such a mistake, and for sure no one becomes a professional by skipping this step. There is no way around it, procrastination is a challenge for me and there are reasons why I duck possibilities for change, especially when I am just about to take a few steps forward. It seems clear where this path will end.

Brooks and Goldstein (2015, p. 16) urge us to assume personal control as a responsibility in order to be happy and resilient: "Taking ownership of our behavior and becoming more resilient requires us to recognize we are authors of our lives." They also posit that "we must not seek happiness by asking someone else to change, but instead always ask what that we can do differently to change the situation?" Retracing the usual way doesn't excite me, so what can I do to be happier and more satisfied? And when? Timing also matters. I cannot decide to start a diet right after a meal, or decide to be brave and further explore the river, once I am back home and the boat is stored in the garage. Tomorrow won't do because as Apollo would shout: "There is no tomorrow!"[13]. I guess changing moments happen in the here and now. As for Rocky, when scared and hopeless, he watched himself in the mirror and realized he had a crossroad in front of him. Apollo's provocation worked, and I

---

[13] This line refers to the sports drama movie *Rocky III* in which the main character Rocky, after badly losing his world title, accepts to be trained by his former opponent Apollo in order to regain his title.

believe any new behavior or change needs some kind of trigger or provocation.

Unlike Rocky, I am not supported by epic and motivational music, but even without a soundtrack I see myself in front of a mirror with a choice to make. Magnum eventually never wrote his investigator's manual, so here and now I ask myself, which kind of pro do I want to be? A procrastinator who keeps going into loops skipping opportunities to improve, or a professional committed in using his experiences to learn, in taking control and responsibility for his personal and professional growth? I feel that somehow in this little airplane chair I can pause from the assault of many routines and take a moment to think about authorship and responsibility for the destination I will pursue. How sweet it would be to have smoother life changes!

For some reason, this reminds me of my regular holidays in Tuscany. Ten days every year, I could finally accomplish one of my dreams: swimming first thing in the morning. Over the years, I've built a routine of 20-25 minutes swimming along a sequence of buoys. This routine energized me and made me feel good, till one day, out of the blue, the lifeguard on board of his water-bike decided that I needed this and that equipment for my safety and visibility. His consideration surprised me, but after years of the same practice, I was not convinced of his point and did not comply until sometime later he reminded me again. That very day, I simply went the other direction along the free beach, away from any supervision. I discovered in this way a nicer area to swim, but most of all, in a few days, without any particular effort, I started to swim two, three, even four times more. How could I cover a longer distance with less effort I do not know. Maybe I was driven by a little resentment, or maybe I felt simply freer in the absence of buoys and established routine. Anyway, I felt something work inside me. I learned something without any reasoning but, nevertheless, I applied it at once smoothly, naturally without conscious awareness. I know I am not talking of a sensational performance, but this little event improved my holidays for the better with more amusement and satisfaction. How joyful it would be to always have such favorable results in such a short time!

I guess we can achieve certain progress silently and without any conscious effort, but what to do when the opposite keeps happening? When, with all possible excitement, we aim for a new direction and, after circling around a bit, end up with the same unsatisfying results? After a few repetitions that lead to identical outcomes, could we expect to change and obtain something different without studying and expanding our knowledge on the matter? Could we aim for a different destination without acquiring new travel instruments and more updated tools?

8.1. *Procrastination*

Einstein said something like, "insanity is doing the same thing over and over again, and expecting different results." I don't want to contradict Einstein, but there is one part to add, since repeating "old, ineffective patterns of behavior despite repeated failures" can be trauma-related, but it is also a consequence of our nature (Cozolino, 2016, p. 8).

A long time ago, Janet (van der Kolk 2000, p. 11) documented that when people are exposed to traumatic events, they experience emotions "too vehement to be integrated." Janet also observed that those memories "were split off from everyday conscious and voluntary control" and "tended to return not as stories of what happened but they were reenacted in the form of intense formal reactions, aggressive behavior, physical pain and bodily states (Ibid). Their separation from awareness "eroded the psychological energy of these traumatized patients." This in turn interfered with the capacity to engage in focused action and learn from the experience. As Freud said, the person is obliged to repeat elements of the past instead of remembering it (Ibid, p. 12). I think I caught something important here. Let me write it down:

Integration of our experiences into conscious awareness allows us to exert voluntary control over them, expand our knowledge and develop more capabilities. On the other hand, non-integrated episodes in our lives limit our possibilities and gain control over us through repeated behaviors.

How relevant is this to my reasoning? Basically, we need to increase awareness or explicit knowledge of our experiences in order to be healthier and I think happier. I also believe there is another consideration: in repeating ourselves, there is a certain level of comfort, a basic level of safety, while change is scary. This is probably why I keep accumulating experiences, words and thoughts without organizing them through writing. Writing pulls me out of the repetition and my comfort zone. It implies being out there and standing up for our ideas and to be vulnerable to critics and unpleasant feedback.

I get it: protection is one reason for procrastination. No, actually it is the other way around. I can see now that procrastination for me is not a consequence of laziness or lack of organization, but a way to protect myself from the fear of the unknown, the discomfort of stepping out of my secure zone and facing vulnerability. What an effective mechanism! It does not require any effort or conscious process, and without damaging my self-image, ensures the final result. A simple "tomorrow" or "later" will keep me on the track of what I consider safe and comfortable without introspection and question marks.

It is brilliant, and maybe it is a pity I do not own the patent of this strategy. Actually, I am quite sure I am not the only one staying at ease on the beaten track. I am not alone in being cuddled by the stream that leads you along the known and verified landscape. In fact, in our long history of evolution, we inherited the potential to develop many extraordinary abilities but also strong and rigid predispositions like choosing safety over all. We are very complex and also delicate organisms, and not everything works as smoothly as it should. Lack of integration of experiences can also happen without past trauma, and leads to the same tendency to repeat our untold/unintegrated stories. Cozolino (2016, p. 7) explains that through our long evolution our brains "have become a patchwork of old and new systems with different languages, operating systems, processing speeds" and I would add, agendas. Since we are this complex of brain functions, and made of very different components, we struggle to coordinate them, with the consequence that we are so vulnerable to "dysregulation, dissociation, and errors in thinking and judgment" (Ibid). He talks of a fast primitive system and a more developed, slow one. Following Siegel's house metaphor they are the ground floor and the first floor.

The difference in processing the information among these two systems creates a gap that, according to Cozolino (2016), explains why so many of us "continue in old, ineffective patterns of behavior despite repeated failures" (p. 8). So here we are: repetition can be a common occurrence due to a communication accident, a "byproduct of our evolutionary history" (Ibid, p. 12).

Einstein, I am not insane after all. Our systems are supposed to self-organize[14] toward integration, but as a matter of fact, they are not always attuned and working together and this explains why we keep taking the same path even though we do not like where it leads. Sailing along the river comes back to my mind and here I am on the boat geared up to enjoy the navigation and ready to explore new ways. Meanwhile while my most evolved part is looking around, feeling contemplative and absorbed in his reasoning, the primitive part, being super-reactive and fast, takes the tiller. So, this is the processing gap in action. The primitive me does not ask or inquire, it just feels and reacts. He gets control as soon as he can and leads toward what he considers to be safer and easier. At the same time, the most evolved component, who considers himself to be the captain of the boat and as such in charge, is turned into a passive passenger in the blink of an eye. At the end of the journey, the captain has no choice but to dock the ship at the usual berth and postpone for some other time any other route or adventure he had mind. The primitive and the most evolved parts are supposed to

---

[14] According to Interpersonal Neurobiology, human brains as complex systems tend to be self-organizing, and move naturally toward integration. They have a driving force to move from simplicity to complexity unless there are internal or external constraints (Bodenoch, 2008).

work in perfect harmony as one, but sometimes this just doesn't happen.

Evolution has led to a hierarchy in which the more evolved should rule, so how can a captain become a passenger? Did he realize what happened? Is he aware that from time to time somebody else jumps in and assumes control? A metaphor is when you are watching TV without paying attention, and somebody else takes control of the remote and changes the program. He does this so many times that eventually you believe you are watching what you intended to.

Following this metaphor, the famous lines from Robert Frost[15] could be rewritten in this way: "Two roads diverged, and without even realizing it, I took the usual one that brought me exactly where I'd left a long time ago." Vertical integration process! This is the point. The entire metaphor speaks to me about the problems that might arise between the two floors of the house. Vertical integration is the way through which the subcortical and cortical areas communicate and allow us to be aware of our body experience and to manage high levels of tension through cortical modulation. It is the way we can escape our reactivity and can become intentional, putting a space between stimulation and reactivity as Vygotsky said (1978, p. 40). And this is just the beginning, since wellbeing, social relationships and any other result I can think of requires this process to function properly. The pure and simple truth is that we have a part of our constitution that is not very conservative but also extremely reactive and gives its best under the radar of our awareness, and for this it is critical that I learn more about it. Let's play with the pencil and see what comes out...

---

[15] The famous lines from Robert Frost are: "Two roads diverged in a wood, and I took the one less traveled by, and that has made all the difference" (Poetry Foundation, 2021b).

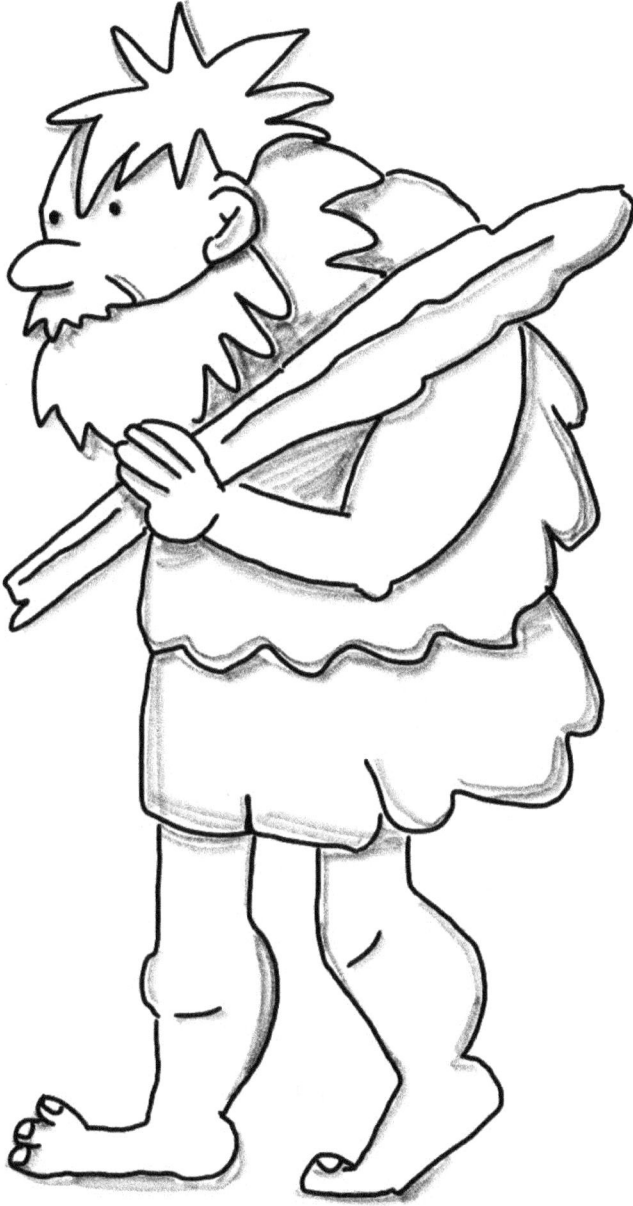

Fig. 3: Primo.

Figure 3 shows Primo and this is his fact sheet:

- Name: Primo (means "first" in Italian) as primitive, because it is the first to be born, and being superfast, he always arrives first (*primo*);

- He grew up before the other system and, for this reason, he feels responsible for both. Survival is his task;

- Primo never sleeps;

- Being primitive, he is super-conservative. Safety is his priority and this is why he refuses to take unnecessary risks. The usual is better;

- As his ancestors, he carved in stone what he knows and believes;

- He continuously collects information, but does not change ideas easily;

- He has well developed senses. He can hear, smell and perceive something the other cannot;

- He is very persistent in having his way. He thinks he is always right: "We are alive after all, aren't we?"

- Primo doesn't know verbal language. He knows a lot, but he communicates exclusively through emotions and bodily sensations;

- He is not stronger, and allows himself to be guided, but you should learn how. If he feels threatened, it is much harder to guide him or to calm him down;

- His agenda is very clear and he never loses his perspective. No distractions for him.

Having made his acquaintance, I have realized a few more things. Exchanging with Primo is not automatic. It takes work to make his implicit knowledge and communication explicit, and practice can improve and strengthen this exchange. This is why after several years I agree with Maureen now: personal psychotherapy for mental health professional is a must.

Primo is not a fierce warrior ready to fight dinosaurs. When scared, he can act as a very small child withdrawing from everything, and everything but the threat disappears. These general conclusions are just a start, so one important task is to get to know him better. I am sure all primitives are similar, but not the same. They have common mechanisms but also unique triggers and maneuvers.

Anyway, there is a constant exchange between our systems at some level, and this determines how we direct our life and expand our abilities. In other words, improving this vertical integration can be an advantage for each and everyone. It is amusing to image a conversation like, "How are you? And how is your old system doing? Pardon me, I forgot her name. Has she been able to have her needs met recently? Very well, mine resents my new job and has been quite activated ever since." Probably this is not an ideal topic of casual conversation, but still it could be a great exercise to expand our awareness on the subject. Having a smooth and attuned relationship among our different brain systems is essential for our wellbeing, and is a necessary requirement for me in my professional capacity of carrying through the intervention we are going to start. I cannot afford to become a passenger along the way, ignoring what to do and where to go. If I want to be a member of a rescue unit, either skipper or sailor, this kind of work requires me to be in charge of my part and to be aware of my own reactions and be skilled enough to manage them.

As on previous occasions, I feel stuck at the bifurcation of this river, wondering which direction to take and endure. Professional or procrastinator? There are pros to consider in both directions. Let me play with this and see what comes out.

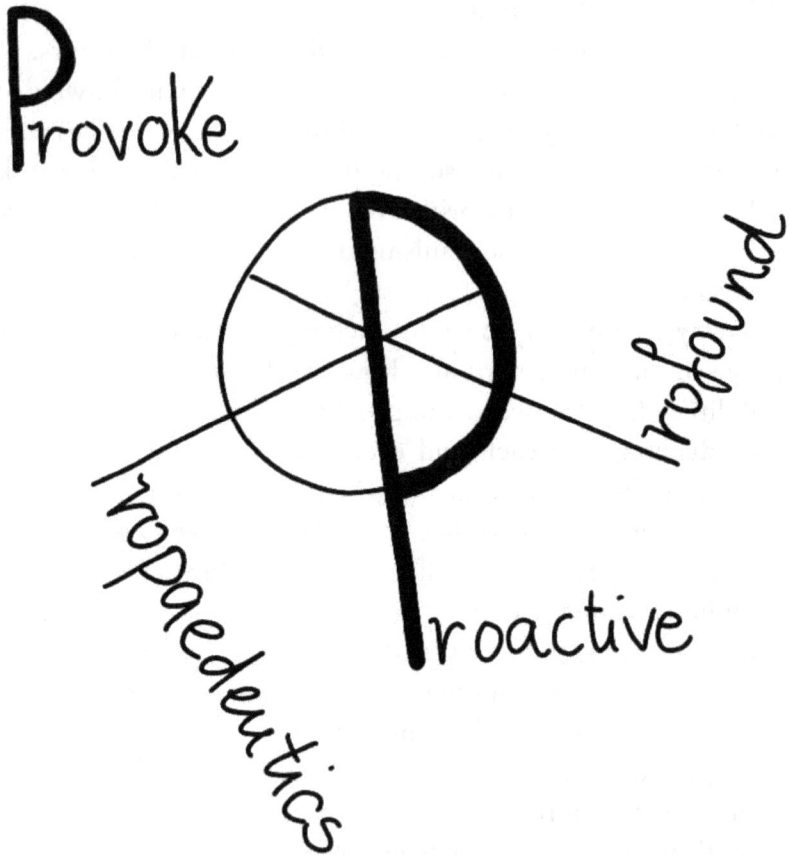

Fig. 4: Provoke, Profound, Proactive, Propaedeutic (clockwise)

When I think of professional, so many pros come to mind. I will keep on playing and try to combine all of them into a single image.

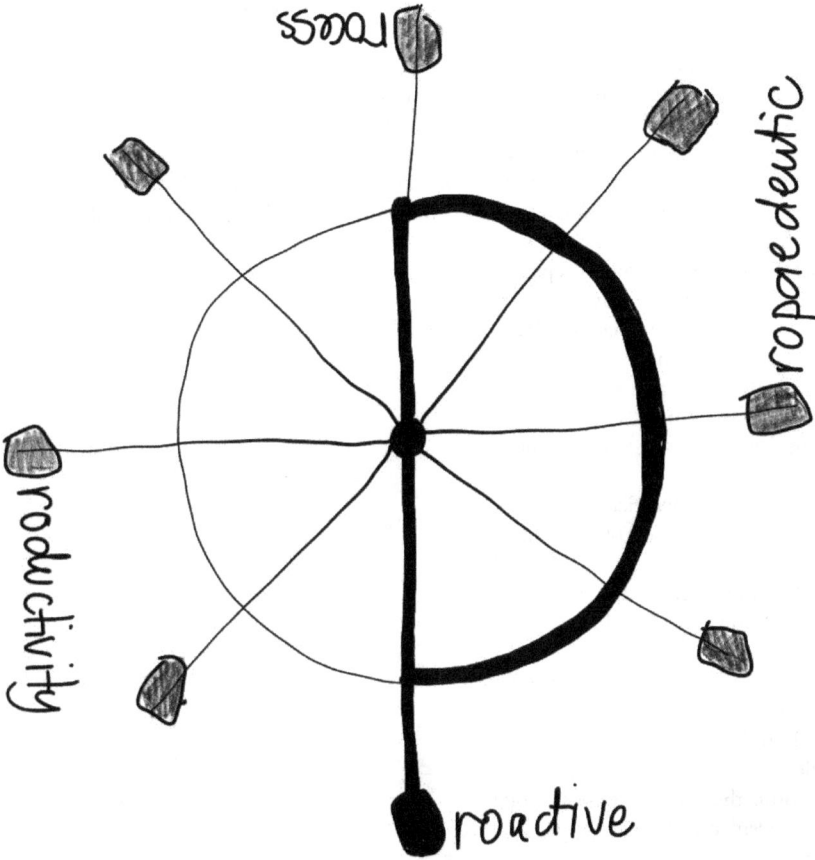

Fig. 5: Process, Propaedeutic, Proactive, Productivity (clockwise from top)

I like this shape (figure 5), it looks harmonious and dynamic. Now I can add some description to fix these ideas.

Professional:	Procrastinator:
Provoke change: do something to trigger or initiate any new path.	**Procrastinate:** elegant strategy to remain in the comfort zone as long as possible.
Proactive: aimed at researching and applying new knowledge and abilities for professional and self development. It requires a constant level of attention and initiative.	**Protection:** the defense from possible risks and problems.
Propaedeutic: "the knowledge necessary before, or for the learning of, a discipline, but not which is sufficient for proficiency"[16]. It refers to the necessary groundwork and preparation required to achieve any goals. It includes also the activities of planning and programming.	**Protest:** active stance to avoid changes and new directions. Using resistance to prevent possibly fearful, painful and discomforting situations.
Profound: the deep and not immediately available content (implicit) of our experience that must be searched and retrieved.	**Probability:** leaving to chance the possibility of reaching interesting results even without full commitment. There is always a likelihood.
Process: the actual practice of exploring and making available implicit knowledge.	
Proceed: taking action by using all available knowledge, including the most profound.	
Proper: the ethical and 'feel right' consideration for which a professional should be prepared as much as possible.	
Progression: the realistic expectation on advancement. It needs to be gradual.	
Proficiency and **productivity:** professional expertise, satisfaction and favorable results. Those are direct consequences of a proactive attitude, constant preparation and profound work.	
Progress: personal improvement and development. It is also a direct consequence of all the previous *pros.*	

Table 1: Professional and procrastinator.

---

[16] The citation refers to the definition indicated at https://en.wikipedia.org/wiki/Propaedeutics (Wikipedia 2020).

8.2. Professional

Part I. Proactive—Enjoy it as a boy, and play it as a grownup

I should probably honor the part of me inclined to choose safety and comfort over the rest, but if I want to be a professional, there is only one direction to take. It is a new course that involves being proactive with considerations, doubts, and knowledge to dig out. I was not aware of myself turning down opportunities to learn and grow and that my procrastination and lack of organization served a purpose. Why I am surprised after all? I should have considered another element together with Primo: the way our internal guidebook is made.

The storage in our brain where we keep all our information and the knowledge that guides us every single moment has a special constitution since it is made of two parts: right and left. These parts are connected and communicate constantly, but they differ in their language and way of operating. The left is composed of words and it is quite easy to consult. The right one is the most up-to-date part on the facts of the world, but organizes its record as body memories, all of it recorded in a nonverbal way. "These are the memories that we do not consciously remember, but never forget (Cozolino 2016, p. 8). They are the wordless stories Damasio talks about, the tracks of our experience of the world, filled of facts and assumptions that prompt us on what to expect and how to behave.

Fantastic! Just to make it easier, during every single moment of our life, we process, store and learn a lot of data without conscious awareness. I need a break or maybe a snack since I keep following so many trains of thoughts. No, I cannot give up to any distractors now, the clock is ticking and the destination is closer.

In my mind, the way I combine these thoughts and psychological theories makes a lot of sense, and this internal Q/R is almost fun. But to make a good use of my time, I have to stop playing and see if I can make something of this because it is very much related to my work. So, now is the moment to add the boring part: the work of refinement. I like what Marvin Hagler said: "Enjoy your activity as a boy and play it as grownup[17]" (Katz, 1981). This means for me that I have to organize and structure my thoughts as if I were speaking with a very patient person. If he or she resisted this point, now it would be perfect to say: "Summarizing, my points are as follows":

1. Our nature

Even as evolved creatures, we maintain a very strong conservative and reactive nature, it is part of our heritage. This component cannot be changed, but it is possible to learn how to communicate with it and guide it.

We are very intelligent creatures, and we use our knowledge to guide our actions all the time. A large part of what we know and learn is implicit. This is the information we receive every millisecond. Even though the contents are not recorded in words and not immediately available to our awareness, they are not secret and can be expressed and somehow decoded.

2. Life events

Stressors are part of our life. Everyone faces difficulties and concerns on a daily basis. There is no safety forever anywhere, but rather we constantly need to make adjustments. We coexist with difficult situations and we regularly adjust to face them. Nevertheless, "prolonged, severe, unpredictable" circumstances (Perry, 2013) can overcome our capabilities and become intolerable. This situation can trigger our primitive part on a permanent basis and lead us in a profound and chronic state of reaction that can be maladaptive at various levels such as cognition, emotions, behavior, neurophysiology and physiology. Then we have traumatic experiences that are tsunamis or powerful recurrent waves that shock and

---

[17]   The citation has been slightly adapted. The real phrase the famous boxer pronounced in an interview with the *New York Times* was: "Enjoy your activity as a boy and play it as a man."

overwhelm everything we hold dear, scattering our beliefs and draining our hopes and sense of power and control in life.

3. Crisis intervention goals

Very often, circumstances cannot be changed and the effort should focus on extending individual and support system resources and possibilities, having in mind the following simple outline:

> Intervention of professionals
> + Individual capabilities
> + Opportunities and life choices
> = Improving quality of life

4. Professionals involved in crisis intervention

Last but not least, the professional working in crisis contexts shares the same human nature as any other person and is not immune to the impact of any life events. Consequently, we have to be very familiar with the points 1, 2 and 3.

This consideration reminds me of a group of paraprofessionals I had to cooperate with almost twenty years ago in Italy, when a terrible earthquake destroyed several villages. The worst feature was that it killed twenty-seven children of the same class, together with their teacher and two other women. I was there from the very first day with different groups of rescuers trained in psychological first aid. We were a disaster response team who had done a lot of previous preparation.

After a month, I received information that a new group of professionals from another branch of the same association had to be part of our intervention. I understood they had some basic psychological knowledge and had learned some field techniques. Our units were a small part of a big machine, and if I wanted to continue coordinating this intervention, I had to adapt to this political decision. A month passed, and for those who had lost their beloved, nothing changed since that terrible October 31st when time stopped. The clock in the main square still indicated *11:32*. For the rescuers, however, this lapse of time had considerably changed working conditions, since the camps were organized and the shifts were now regular and predictable. With the new group, the discussion started by phone and continued once they were at our camp. They wanted to practice psychological first aid and so their boss called me several times.

They were not aware of how slow and delicate the process is to build up relationships before applying any techniques in a crisis context. They ignored the need for the helper to adapt to the survivor's needs and not the other way around, and, more generally, they neglected everything that needs to precede even the best practice.

That day, the afternoon seemed endless, filled with inconclusive talking. Everyone was still repeating his lines when we got the information that three members of the group felt sick. Their coordinator and I reached the same conclusion: they were physically reacting to the situation. Even though they hadn't had the opportunity to meet or speak with any survivors yet, staying in the camp was enough to perceive the pain and despair in the air. Their condition was too strong to be ignored and their coordinator was sensitive and reasonable enough to realize that we all needed to be more careful. Together we redefined their contribution to the project, starting with practical activities. We made the process gradual, and considerable group and individual supervision was the first task to protect both survivors and rescuers. Eventually, the new group was fully integrated too and had the chance to prove to be of great help.

Part II. Propaedeutic—Setting sails

I had almost forgotten this episode, but it proves once more that in this area of work, theory does not count much without other key elements. Too often, the preparation of professionals who want to commit themselves to this work is focused merely on technicalities while other important aspects are left aside. Examples are: how to improve the knowledge of our personal "reactive side," and how to learn to relate with it? How to make the best use of our knowledge (implicit and explicit) in our work? How to develop awareness in the role of our internal guidebook in leading our behavior and, finally, how to learn to elaborate our wordless experience of the day and even of the moment?

This has little or nothing to do with stress management and self-care standard courses, but is much wider and is related with preparing ourselves to be authors of our own life. In this regard, it makes a lot of sense what Cozolino (2016) says, the primary function of the psychotherapist is "to teach clients that not only can they edit their present story, but they can also be authors of new stories" (p. 16). How could we possibly help others if we are not committed in this process first? Surely we cannot sort out all the elements of this journey without preparing ourselves. It is gradual and progressive work. Nobody becomes a professional athlete on the day of the competition, by training just on Sundays or watching others competing. There is necessary prior knowledge, the only thing that can be achieved in a short time is the determination to be more and more prepared. This is step one: know the direction you want to go. Speaking of directions, for some reason George Gray's poem in the *Spoon River Anthology* comes to mind (Masters, 2007, p. 39):

> I have studied many times
> The marble which was chiseled for me—
> A boat with a furled sail at rest in a harbor.
> In truth it pictures not my destination
> But my life. (...)
> I hungered for meaning in my life.
> And now I know that we must lift the sail
> And catch the winds of destiny
> Wherever they drive the boat.

Working in crisis contexts requires, more than in other professions, to expect the unexpected, to sail in unknown and troubled waters. Crisis has the power to disrupt personal stories and life paths, imposing often rigid new lines. It is a storm that can cast you away, damage your sails or make you scared of the sea forever. After you suffer such experiences, time stops and the wish or strength to go on vanishes. Our very nature and the vehemence of events can make it very tempting also for professionals to remain safe in harbor, uttering easy thoughts of wisdom from the docks. But how could we help someone as George Gray if we *are* Gray too? "Look George, my boat is safe and guarded in the harbor, but you can sail the wind of destiny if you wish." Could it work? Would it work for me? Who would I rather trust instead? If I had to plan an expedition to a remote and difficult location, who would I choose as consultant? A tourist who just got off from his round trip across the lake, a wanderer who has been in places and has a lot of tales to share, or a researcher, somebody who spends his life exploring? This tripartition comes back again, so let me write it down, since I could use it somewhere.

The Tourist, the Wanderer and the Researcher

The Tourist

There are many kinds of tourists, with different ideas of vacations, but all of them are driven by the wish to enjoy new or well-known locations. The tourist might also be very passionate about these visits or activities. Nevertheless, the experiences are always time-limited. The holiday ends at some time, and the tourist goes back home to his usual life with a bag of happenings and probably the desire for other holidays. Travel and visits could be a relevant part of this person's life, but they remain complementary and temporary activities as other pastimes might be.

The Wanderer

The life of the wanderer is dedicated to traveling, visiting places and collecting different experiences. He follows his instinct and interests in choosing the destination as he adapts to contingent situations. His bag can be rich with experiences and findings, but those are not collected and organized by using a predefined method. He might be passionate about exploring, but pursuing specific objectives is never his first goal. He travels for the sake of the experience.

The Researcher

He is driven by a well-defined purpose. The exploration is highly organized and goal-oriented. The researcher is fully committed in the actual process of seeking, but also in the groundwork of setting the most suitable research methodology and the most effective tools. He is ready to take risks and his energy is focused on discovering, but also on keeping track of the route and systematically considering all attempts made.

Part III. Process and proceed—The wind of destiny

Looking at this tripartition, some questions come to my mind: am I tourist, a wanderer or a researcher? Where do I locate myself? What about my own sailing in the open sea? I remember the drawing I did in a training course to represent myself more than two decades ago. It was a boat sailing along the coast. I also recall that no more than half an hour ago I was metaphorically stuck at the bank of a river and I changed direction almost as soon as I started to explore a new path. Not really an impeccable research vessel.

Being generous with myself, I should acknowledge that I found something, even if accidentally. Some implicit concepts became explicit and, as in a proper process of integration, they became "flexible elements of the decision making and not anymore unconscious determinants" (Bodenoch, 2008). I wasn't aware of my procrastination pattern, and through the metaphor and the writing I realized how I deal with trying to do something new. I would not say it is a full process or a proper research expedition, but it is a start. Procrastination and postponing prevent changes and help Primo to relax. This doesn't qualify as deep research, since it is probably common to all mankind.

Primo, my friend, I know what I am doing. As a professional, I have the responsibility to expand my search and know more about my guidebook and get to know more about my own story. Even for athletes, training is only a part of their preparation, and I forget too often that I have a body that accumulates stories to tell, and wisdom to use. So I will start focusing on the section where the wordless

stories are, and I will use symbols to give them a voice. As stories
described by art pieces or music, these cannot be translated straight
into words either. For instance, what is the translation into words of
Bach's Cello Suite Number 1, or Vivaldi's Four Seasons? Their contents are deeper and wider than just a title, and must be expressed
first and only then analyzed. For this reason, I will use the tools I
have available here: metaphors and drawings. Let's keep exploring. I
am going to start from the image of me in a canoe taking the small
tributary on the side instead of my usual course on the main river.

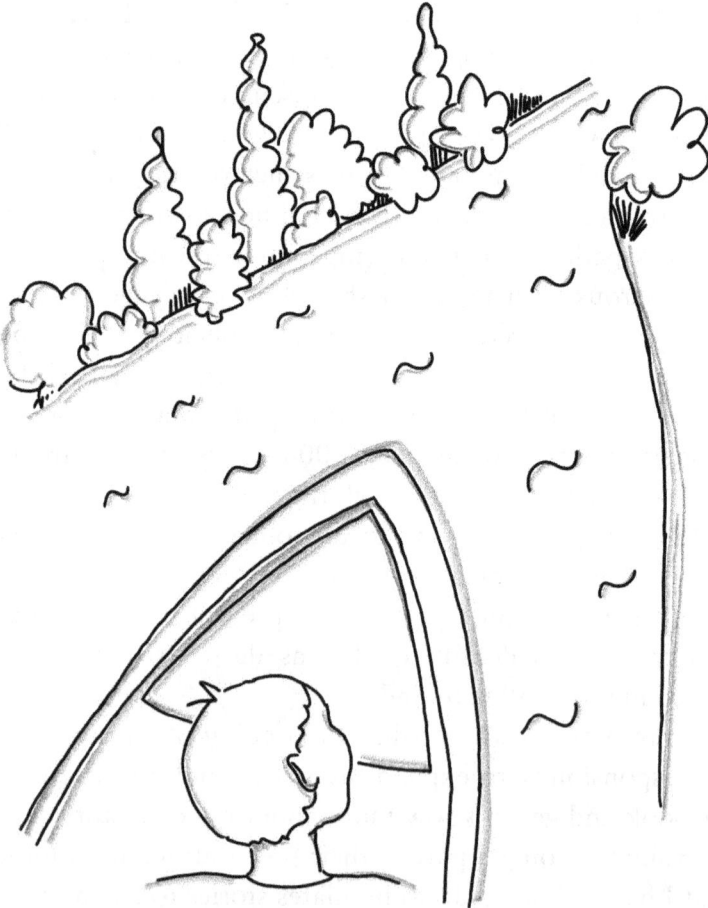

Fig. 6: Claudio in a canoe going down a small tributary

I do not even need to write any words about this drawing. Simply imagining myself in this new direction with the river behind me, I feel a succession of emotions. A moment of pure joy and excitement is soon replaced by a sentiment of sorrow, an indefinite sense of pain for leaving something behind. It is only a sketch, and yet these lines drawn on paper evoke real, strong feelings.

I realize that proceeding and going on, although exciting, somehow makes me feel that I am leaving something back and this hurts me. Now I truly understand the saying "leaving is a little like dying." Taking new ways is leaving at least habits, which affects older parts of us. It is painful and can raise strong resistance. No wonder it is so hard to move on to explore. Dwelling on these words, I realize that the drawing I recalled a few minutes ago finally makes sense. It is the drawing in which I depicted myself as a boat along the coast. Keeping this metaphor in mind, the following lines come to my mind:

My boat did not have "furled sail at rest in a harbor." In fact, I sailed and navigated a lot, but up and down along the coast. I feared the open sea. I did not lift up my sails to fully catch the wind of destiny and if I did at one point, I turned back because I felt I'd gone too far. I reefed the sails for the sadness of leaving something I was attached to.

The moral to this metaphor now is more complete and it is something like: if I go too far, I have to leave my beloved behind. Part of my story says that departures across the sea cause suffering to me and to people I love. This process has shed surprising light on how my past experiences have reinforced this conservative attitude that despises departures and long explorations. Traveling, exploring, working in distant contexts has never been smooth, but always involved pain to deal with and negotiation between different parts of me. I've probably always felt the conflict between opposing needs and beliefs, but I've never put it into words like today. I lived with the deep conviction that moving on creates suffering. but even though it was hard, I did move on and sailed away, and I long for more of it. How often these words from Whitman (Poetry Foundation, 2021a) have echoed in my mind:

Still here I carry my old delicious burdens,

I carry them, men and women, I carry them with me wherever I go,

I swear it is impossible for me to get rid of them.

Part IV. Productivity and progression—The sea of possibilities

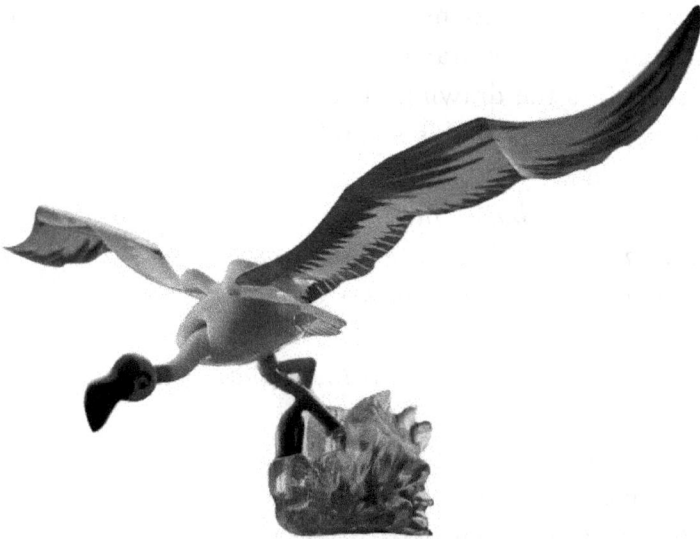

Fig. 7: A trapped bird

Perhaps it is my suggestibility, but I can see a kind of message in the small miniature found in a chocolate egg (Figure 7). I watch this bird and it comes to my mind that our nature and past experience can be a block, a trap that prevents us from moving forward, and yet at the same time it can become a springboard that helps us to fly. Hey bird, do you feel trapped, or you are ready to spread your wings?

It is so true that "history is not destiny" (Cohen, 1990), and if we can't undo and erase our past, as Cozolino (2016) suggests, we might add more verses and new chapters. I cannot say for certain, but as our evolving brain develops and improves, adding pieces to old historical parts, we also thrive in the same way. As in the history of mankind, the mammalian and cortical brain were built on the reptilian structure extending human capabilities, and our personal stories work in a similar fashion. We do not erase our past, we do not put the clock back, but we expand and update our living knowledge and capabilities. Through a long process, we extend our available resources to embrace a new direction and even to travel new and fulfilling paths.

The last written lines can give a whole new meaning to the entire story; they can be the springboard! So, here are a few taking points:

Processing (as an operation that allows implicit knowledge to become explicit) extends our knowledge, resources and capabilities. We become more aware of the "narrative arcs of our life story and this helps us to understand that alternative story lines are possible" (Cozolino, 2016, p. 16). In this way, we acquire new information and tools for navigating, but the actual sailing, the real change, requires one more step: the courage to take consistent action. This is "*proceed*," move further with what you have understood. Set your instruments and then go, use your knowledge and tools for taking charge of writing how you want the story to continue.

I know processing and proceeding may generate pain and a lot of protest, but eventually it opens the way to more possibilities. In this way, we can set the sail and open ourselves to the risk of the unknown, but also to new opportunities. New landscapes and new lines can add to our story. Wait a moment, here it is! The same framework that applies to crisis intervention applies perfectly also to anyone who wants to change and improve his life.

> *Process/intervention*
> *+ Individual capabilities (more knowledge and resources available)*
> *+ Opportunities and life choices*
> *= Improve quality of life*

Certainly it is a simplified framework that does not take into account the complexity of many situations, but it has the advantage of providing a perspective. More resources become available as knowledge and skills result in more opportunities. Using them (proceeding) consistently leads to an improved life. For instance, improved ability in recognizing and facing stressors makes life easier. In addition, supporting other people in expanding their self-awareness gives them more opportunities to be in charge of the direction of the change they want to make in life. So, I have to adapt the chart:

Process/intervention	
+ Individual capabilities (more knowledge and resources available)	*Feeling in charge: individuals can navigate forward, "write other chapters"*
+ Opportunities and life choices	*choose the direction they want to take and*
= Improve quality of life	*proceed*

> The final result is individuals being authors of their own improvement so they can write additional chapters that give a different meaning to the entire story.

Fig. 8: Process/Intervention Model

This chart integrates perfectly with the approach CPBF. This is why we need our MAP to be clear and our program to be flexible enough to provide the space for individuals and communities for self-direction as authors of their own life.

Considering a previous metaphor of writing a play by performing it, I could also say that our scope in crisis intervention is supporting individuals and communities to be script writers, stage builders and actors of their own "theater." Our responsibility as professionals is to co-construct the stage where people can uncover their past stories and decide which future plays they want to perform, and then to support their acting. Being a resource in this process requires professional construction capacities, but also the personal ability to *read* our own past stories, *write* new chapters, and *act* them. How could it be possible to contribute to any play without the abilities of *reading, writing* and *acting*? Here we are, another way to say that I cannot escape from process and proceed. MAP and experiences are fundamental for this work but are not enough.

I think I did my part today. I *read* in my past so far that I fear the open sea, I *wrote* that I am ready to move on and set sails risking the pain in order to gain further possibilities. Now is the moment to *act*, and I have decided that the best way for me is stay focused on writing the notes on self-care. Perfect, coping with present while building for the future.

Final notes

Any changes must be provoked, initiated and proactively supported. Specific results require a propaedeutic part, a preparation. An essential aspect of this groundwork both for professionals and for their clients includes expanding and using the implicit profound personal knowledge we all have. All this delicate and hard work might not bring the results we aim for, but sets us on the way to expand our possibilities and life opportunities. This improves both our current life and our future prospects, and puts us in charge of our path. Our last line has the potential to define our entire story.

9 Self-Care: Before, During and After a Crisis Intervention

The last part of core training is very important; it does not only refer to crisis intervention, but also includes the period before and after it. Some years ago, when I was fancying to write a book on crisis settings, I thought the last chapter should be dedicated to self-care. I also imagined the title: *Buckle up.* I had in mind the image of fastening a seatbelt before departure as a way of representing the need to ensure our own safety. With time, I realized that this metaphor emphasizes quite a passive role. More recently, I thought that a boxing analogy would be more appropriate. "Protect yourself at all times" is what the referee tells the athletes before the match. In boxing, the act of defense is a very active stance: in addition to using your arms as shields, you duck, anticipate, manage the distance, etc. Nevertheless, this is still not enough. What does each of us need in order to work in very difficult situations? And how can we be sure to have what we need when we need it? I believe this is a matter of advance preparation, and practicing self-care skills regularly. We cannot demand an instant beach body just because today we decided to go to the seaside for our holidays.

Sometimes we might find habits or activities that work perfectly for us even without any conscious effort. I think of my father. In the last period of his life, he had a health condition that restricted his movements and routines a lot. Even so, some time every day, helped by my mother and his stick, he put on his sunglasses and said with a big smile, "I am going on a cruise," and then moved outside to the balcony. Sitting on his chair, he gazed at the dance of the clouds and the flight of the birds and, even though the view was not fantastic, he looked calm and appreciative as if he were really admiring a beautiful panorama. This was an excellent self-care routine. Nothing studied, planned or thought could have worked better. I don't know how he got there, but he found what he needed just at the right moment. I wish we all could find something similar to *cope with the present* in the toughest times. However, a professional with responsibility for others should consider also the additional step of *building for the future*, working on something that might be useful and applicable also in different and forthcoming circumstances.

I think self-care should consider a proactive process that involves preparation before fieldwork, management on the job, and a self-care plan after that. I will start the module with this quote, which is useful to raise curiosity and lead us in the exploration of the subject:

"Stories also serve as powerful tools for neural network integration. The combination of a linear storyline and visual imagery woven together with verbal and nonverbal expressions of emotion activates circuitry of both cerebral hemispheres, cortical and subcortical networks, the various regions of the frontal lobes, the hippocampus, and the amygdala" (Cozolino, 2016, p. 15).

Since we have talked about stories, I am going to share with you a personal embarrassing experience on TV. I still remember the cameraman, the young journalist and me sitting comfortably at the restaurant where I used to eat with my colleagues. They chose a good spot, with a proper light. I liked their idea of making a documentary on the terrible earthquake in Bam. They wanted to offer a wide perspective, including the role of the psychosocial intervention. I remember I felt at ease and very clear-minded. All of a sudden the journalist asked me: "What has been your most difficult moment so far?" I thought a little, then I answered that it was when I'd met Mr. Mustafa. I started to tell about my encounter with him. At one point, I could not restrain my tears anymore and I cried in front of the camera. What was this encounter about?

I had a problem with the plumbing system in my apartment and, Mr. Mustafa came to fix it. We tried to have a conversation during the time he was there. I knew some words in Farsi and he knew some in English. He was a very composed and elegant person, and he could focus on his work while managing our conversation. When he finished working, on his way out, just outside the apartment doorstep he stopped and said: "Five." I did not understand immediately, so he repeated, showing with his hand the number five.

I did not get it immediately. He meant that he had lost five family members in that earthquake: wife, daughter, mother and two brothers. I can still see him in the darkness outside the door, collecting his tools, and a few moments later disappearing in the night. At that time, he was probably the age I am now, maybe he was younger. After I closed the door and after few seconds I started crying. It felt like a punch in the stomach.

I still do not know what struck me the most, that all the people I was working with had suffered immense losses, but it was like another painful reality was abruptly revealed to me. Mr. Mustafa and I were in the same compound and I had met him every day for two months before this episode, but I had never realized the terrible pain he was carrying. Probably there were signs I could have recognized: he constantly dressed in black, his movements were gentle but very self-restrained, like a person who is carrying the weight of the world on his shoulders; he was mostly alone and had sculpted on his face the expression of a person who has no other choice but to go on. A lot was there, but I could not see it.

Who knows what kind of reactions and thoughts this story can evoke. I started crying in front of a camera, recollecting this memory months later. At the time of the interview, my first thoughts were that I had not worked hard enough on myself. Then I guessed I did not know myself enough. My current belief is that I was not giving myself a proper space to express the stories I was collecting, despite the fact that I was teaching a lot about trauma and referring to the limits of talking when we come to a traumatic reaction. I did not apply my knowledge to myself.

The story I just told is incomplete if I do not add one more piece. In that period, as I do now, I was quite dedicated to self-care: I had a daily routine of physical activities, I was writing a journal, I was taking time for dynamic and static meditation using Qi Gong. I also connected regularly with my family. These were good activities that brought me relief and a general sense of wellbeing, but there was a flaw: they were all attempts in different directions, a constant digging in distinct parts of the landscape, small explorations in various locations. It was like writing different sentences, poems and drawing images and instead of putting all of them together in the same story, scattering them all around. If I think of the powerful experience with Mr. Mustafa, I realize I did not process it. I did not put the pieces of the story together as a coherent whole; in other words I did not integrate them in my autobiographical story.

Self-care has many components. A crucial one is processing experiences. Also, for this topic, there are many theories and approaches to consider. I decided to present you the Right-Left-Right Progression (McGilchrist, 2012).

The first stage of the progression is non-linguistic and it originates in the Right Hemisphere (RH) of the brain, which is the part "more in touch with reality" (Ibid). In the RH, the experience is presented as a non-verbal implicit body memory or, as called by Damasio, a "wordless story" (1999, p. 188).

The Left Hemisphere (LH) of the brain "brings the experience into focus, unpacks the wholeness implicit and makes it explicit and allows it to be formulated in language" (McGilchrist, 2012). The added value is a re-presentation of the world that is more stable and organized. Through this phase, the experience is enriched through conscious, detailed analytic understanding. As a result, the new knowledge is created like the writing of new sentences or paragraphs of a story. But this is a staging post and not the end of the process. In fact, this new part can make sense only if it is inserted into a global story: our autobiographical story.

The third part of the process is the reintegration of the new explicit contents in the realm of the experience in the RH. The reintegration occurs when the new paragraphs that can be integrated in the autobiographic story are expressed through the use of metaphors, *since they are functions of the RH and rooted in the body.*

"What begins in the right hemisphere's world is sent to the left hemisphere's world of processing, but must be returned to the world of the right hemisphere where a new synthesis can be made" (McGilchrist, 2012).

To summarize, the first part of the process (the non-linguistic) is what happens naturally when we live an experience. At this stage we are the "patient recipient;" at the second stage, we become the "powerful operator" of the experience itself (Ibid). In the third stage, we expand the knowledge about ourselves and the world and we are able to truly learn from the experience.

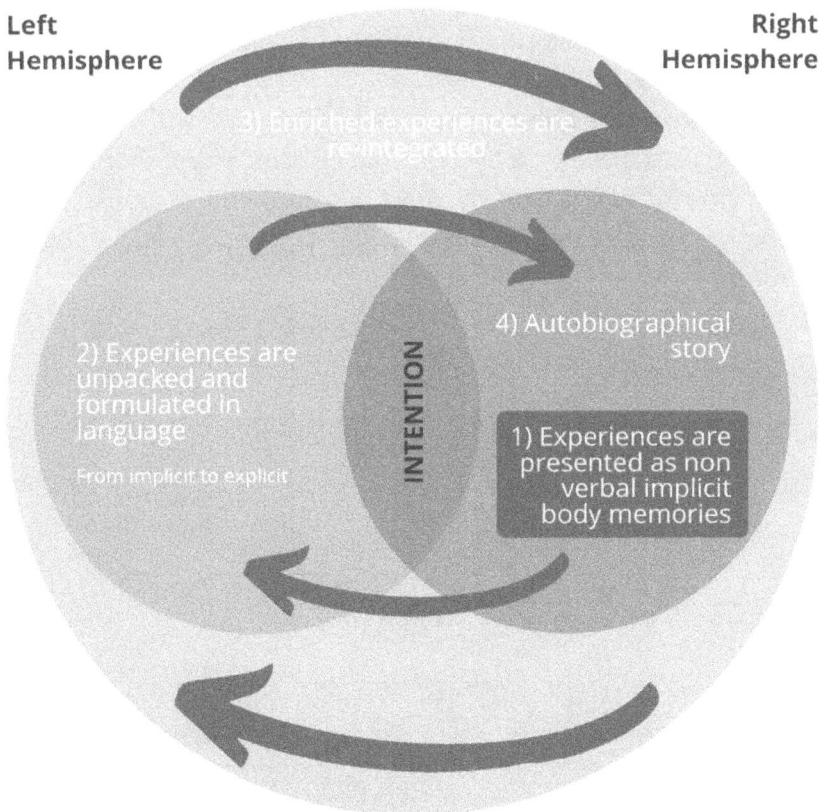

Fig. 9: Right-left-right progression, inspired by McGilchrist (2019).

What I wanted to underline with the previous story is that this progression of phases does not happen automatically and it is not immediate. Our experiences can remain implicit (RH), and also denatured or decontextualized (LH). In the crisis intervention field, it is necessary to be familiar with the integration or re-integration process. The story I shared is now part of my autobiography. In fact, today I am able to tell the facts, to be aware of my own feelings, what it meant for me and what I learned from it. How did I do it?

Humans have common mechanisms, but each of us is unique. Finding the most suitable practice to promote this "progression" is a matter of personal research and consistent intentional exercise. For this reason, to close the session, I would like to suggest that my audience should go through the process, in order to get the idea of how this progression works. *Would you please represent the journey we shared today using the expressive materials at your disposal in this room, including the miniatures?* Afterward, I will invite you to write a story about it on a sheet of paper. *Can you find a metaphor and the title of this story? Is there an aesthetic response (such a drawing or a movement) you would like to produce and share with the group?*

10   The Painter

The hard work of processing made me hungrier. Next time I will add some cheese to the sandwich. I needed almost thirty years to improve my travel, but now I sense I can progress faster. Where is my snack? I could never eat my snack without offering some to my neighbor.

C: "Hi, my nutritionist told me that if I am good in following my diet I can reward myself. Would you like a chocolate egg?"

P: "Yes, thanks. I like them. My name is Pete."

C: "I am Claudio. Is the Island your final destination?"

P: "Yes, I am going to visit my family and I would also like to help."

C: "Is any of your family hurt?"

P: "No, they live in part of the Country where the disaster didn't hit. You know, I am a painter and I have a lot of experience in renovations. I figured I might give a hand."

C: "A painter? You are an artist then. I am very fascinated by painting."

P: "Thank you. I live basically with paints and brushes in my hands, but that doesn't make me an artist. I can say I am a professional though. After so many years, I can do basically any kind of painting. I also like decorating when I am asked to."

C: "Allow me a question even though it might sound silly. I always follow the instructions on the cans on how to prepare the paint but it never works! The combination is always too dense or too liquid even if I am extremely precise. How come?"

P: "Honestly, I don't know how to answer. You see, my technique and the way I paint is almost automatic now and I don't read the instructions. What I do is feeling the paint, the surface and I also know my tools, the different brushes, the quality of the paints."

C: "I see, this is interesting. So, neither I nor the instructions are wrong. How could I improve? Do you have some advice or formula to share with me?"

P: "Probably there are workshops you may take, these days you can find them also online. Personally, I learn by watching others and practicing lots, and now I can say I am able to respond to a client's requests most of the time. I think the most important element is to practice and pay attention to your practice. I don't want to make it complicated, but in this work there is a constant adjustment. There are differences in the surface, the kind of paint, the temperature, the brush, the clients. This is probably the reason why pre-established formulas don't work. I have been painting for twenty years and I always pay attention to what I do. Sometimes I don't realize that I am changing techniques or tools, but other times I have to think about it and plan otherwise."

C: "Pete, there are no shortcuts then. This makes so much sense to me. There are no techniques that work per se. There is always the necessity to feel and adjust. I am a psychologist and I work with families. Can you believe that somebody thinks that with people in disasters, it is possible to apply protocols and standard techniques as if everyone was the same?"

P: "No way, this can't be true! Even windows of a house are not the same. There is exposure to the sun, humidity and type of wood to consider."

C: "I could not agree more. I have wooden windows at home. I painted them several times myself, but all of them look colored by different people with different skills and experience."

P: "Ahaha! Anyway, it is good you practice, and do not experiment in other people's home. You have to know very well what you are doing."

C: "Yes, I like to renovate my home, but I know my limits and I always thought that, unlike amateurs, professionals are able to manage unexpected situations. So when things are complicated, I just hire experts."

P: "You are right *(laughing)*, complex situations sometimes can become even more complex! I think when you are dedicated to a profession, you know how to find solutions when problems arise, and you don't get scared anymore. In the worst scenario, you just pretend you are in control and use your experience to figure out a way to deal with the situation. You know, Claudio, actually I have a secret for a good work: preparation. Before starting any work, take time to think about what to do, all the steps the work requires. Then clear the space around you, choose and organize your material in good order and carefully work the surface you need to paint. It is that investment of time that will save you time eventually and will prevent possible problems. It might be boring, I know, but it creates a good base and helps you to feel more comfortable."

C: "This is great advice. I always forget the action before the action. This makes me think to a sort of Italian proverb '*Ti va l'acqua per l'orto.*' The literal translation is: 'The water goes in your garden,' and it is used to address somebody's luck. The saying underlines that everything is going so well for a person that even though it was not planned, extra water is reaching his garden. I find this proverb very interesting because for me it underlines the importance of preparation more than luck."

P: "I see what you mean, because I have a garden myself. What is considered as 'luck' is instead the reward for work that is not always visible."

C: "Yes, as in your case, good work is the result of different phases. The gardener for instance studies the soil, the inclination of the land, then digs and works the land and the lines to ensure the possibility of collecting water and to directing the flow to reach all the vegetables."

P: "This is the perfect example of groundwork *(laughing)*. It is easy to make holes in the garden, but to prepare the soil and irrigation is something else. Sometimes the neighbor's garden is greener just because he prepares it better."

C: "Good preparation set the base for good results."

P: "I agree!"

C: "I am really glad your family wasn't hurt in the earthquake and I'm sure you will be very helpful to your people."

P: "Thanks. I'll start simply with the tools and resources I have. I took six months off work, so it is a good time for me."

C: "You make me think of one of the best project I have ever seen."

P: "Please, tell me about it."

C: "It was not far from your Island. Do you remember the earthquake in Haiti?"

P: "Sure, my family felt it too."

C: "I worked there for several months and started by making an assessment. I wanted to understand the situation and in which way we could be helpful. At the time, one of the biggest needs for people was to have shelters. In meeting survivors, I noticed that not much was done and I also knew that the biggest organizations were busy in discussing the kind of temporary structure to build. Eventually it took eleven months to decide the kind of shelter to build."

P: "I am not surprised, honestly."

C: "My organization did not have the resources for that, and much later we were able to build just a few ones for community purposes. But in the first stages, I met a group of retired carpenters who really impressed me. They were very aware of the resources, tools, material and abilities they could use. They searched an area where they were allowed to work, and after getting agreement from the land owners, they built wooden shelters just beside the collapsed houses. In two weeks they built six or seven houses. I admired the way they worked, even involving the locals: simple and super effective. I think about them often in the different context of my work."

P: "I have something similar in mind with my cousins. Nothing big, but we'll do our best."

C: "Now I understand what you were drawing before I interrupted you. Shelters and warehouses."

P: "Exactly, I just have to add few details and then I'll figure some numbers. I want to have a clear idea before meeting my cousins."

C: "I have to finish something too. But I am glad we had chance to talk before landing."

P: "Likewise. Give me your address. I'd like to know more about the work you do here, and I can also give you some advice on your future painting adventures if you like!"

C: "I would love both, thanks."

11   Beyond the Clouds

What a temptation, the guy in front of me is watching that intense action movie, *Sicario* or *Soldado*, I don't recall which of the two, but I remember well that scene where two CIA agents meet after a long time and one says to the other, "You should consider investing in sunscreen." What a greeting! Actually, as I see my face reflected in the dull screen before me, I realize that I should have invested more in myself. Definitely the life we conduct shapes our presence. I agree with the saying that looking at our body is like peeking into our past: wrinkles, scars, injuries, the structure of our body, our posture are just a part of it. Experiences modify our body and they also sculpt our brain, and some part of it for good. As McGilchrist (2019, p. 8) wrote, "The past is no more dead than we are because it is something that we perform every living day." He is right. Our brain is not only conservative according to its ancient and primitive constitution, but is also an "historical organ." Our experiences define our network system "making associations between sensory signals co-occurring in any given moment in time" (Perry 2013). These associations are stored as templates that eventually guide our behavior. In this way, the past experiences stored in our guidebook lead our action in the future. It is fantastic because this makes us capable of learning and adapting, but also "vulnerable to being trapped by associations that are irrational, false or have no longer a reason to exist" (Ibid). Now it makes sense what Jung posited: our organs are a museum, our brain reflects the history of mankind and just through the act of creation, we evolve and move forward from mankind and our history (cited in McGilchrist 2019, p. 8). From this perspective, I understand that to escape our history, we are doomed to be creative. Creativity then is not a hobby or a luxury, but a necessity.

I believe on this plane I have done a bit of both: history lessons and attempts to be creative. Since this journey began, I have often repeated certain patterns of behaviors and trains of thought, but it was not an oblivious repetition since I *realized* what was happening. In theatrical terms, I can say that I initially *acted* my old implicit script and, at some point, I became aware of that. The big difference this time is that I was able to *read* the past scripts I was acting (making them explicit) and I decided to *write* new ones and eventually I *acted* them. So, during this journey, I did not just avoid a screen marathon but almost completed all the sequences of a play, a small expression of creativity that directed me onto a different path. This happened because, as McGilchrist (2019, p. 21) would say, instead of reacting I was able to stand back from the world in order to gain control over it. As humans, we have the need to live the moment of our bodily experience and we also have the capacity to get some distance from it. McGilchrist (Ibid) puts it in a beautiful way: on the one side there is the immediate experience, the "terrain" where we engage with the world and, on the other side, as humans we also have the unique capability of moving above it and gaining a wider perspective of the territory. These concepts are the horizontal and the vertical axis.

Forced by the situation, with poor liberty of movement, fewer distractions, and a great and respectful neighbor, I gained verticality. I paused from the terrain, took distance and have seen patterns and different lines of my story re-enacted over and over. I guess each of us finds his pause time in different ways, and this long flight over the ocean worked very well for me. However, I should look for something else, because this practice is obviously too expensive to become regular! In any case, taking off from the terrain is just one step, since having a new perspective is important but not sufficient.

In fact, in this very copybook that I recycled long ago, I still have the notes I took some years back to keep track of my intent to lose weight. I've never looked at them carefully, and I've never ripped them out either and now I know why. For each day there is a line that reports date, weight, amount of time exercising, average heart rate during training and kind of exercise performed. At a glance, the evidence: I was gaining weight almost on a daily basis. The numbers did not lie. Something worked exactly the other way around. Could those pages have been clearer? No. Was that message enough to reverse the results? No. Actually, that was the reason why I gave up the records before the end of the second page, with 5 kg more. The picture gave the verdict, but did not explain the reasons why, and what to do instead. It was a good start, but looking at our history pages is not enough to change them. I missed the creativity component, and needed a deeper look and the act of creating something, a new script to write and play. In technical terms, I missed verticality, processing and proceeding.

Today is different because I took off, but I also moved far and kept flying up where I silenced the terrain and was able to make space for metaphors and images to emerge. And then the real work started, because I played those images and wordless stories and tried to give them voice. I traveled on the *diagonal* axis up and forward beyond the clouds where duties, old and repetitive patterns and the fear of the unknown lost their power and the entire itinerary could be considered. Here is where I met Primo and where I opened the guidebook of repeated stories. From here I could see how far in the past the boat along the coast actually was. I became aware that for years I'd kept identifying with a chapter that belongs to my history. In fact, eventually I sailed away from the coast, moved away from the known through many seas and oceans. It was often painful, but I did reach many different places. My vessel is no more a coastline boat but a sea wanderer that has experienced and learn a lot in the different travels. Yes, it is a wanderer that collected so many short stories with different morals, a lot of which are yet to be completed.

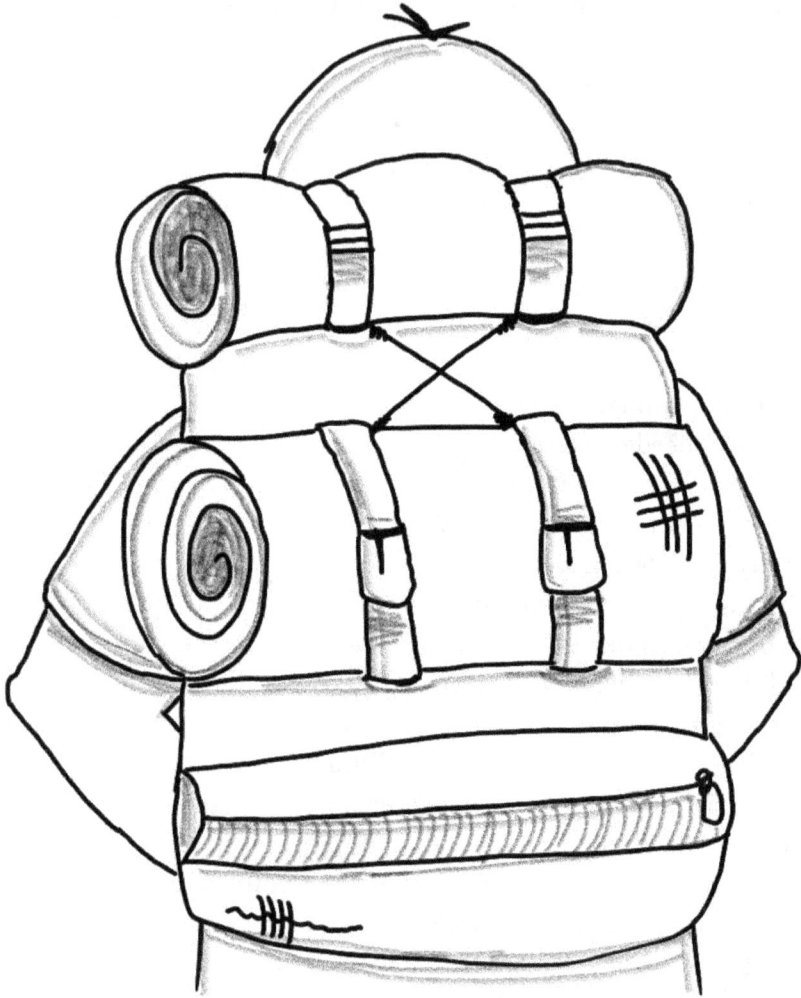

Fig. 10: A backpacker

If I had to draw something to give a shape to this image and express my perceptions, it would be something like a backpacker (Figure 10) who fills his big pack with different objects, notes and pictures. He is eager to collect pieces but seldom reorganizes them.

The moment I saw the first lines on paper, I realized that this is also an old chapter. The images of the backpacker and the sea wanderer no longer apply. They do not represent me anymore. I became more organized, goal oriented, constant in my work and more aware of the different elements that affect my job. Isabella, the deadlines, my own frustration and the different contexts almost forced me to give up wandering. I can't say I arrived at this point quickly, easily or that my quest is ended, but I went far and high enough to realize that in addition to having the proper curriculum for some work, I am also aware of what I can bring into a crisis context. I am more aware than ever that in my bag I no longer have a collection of different notes but a MAP that can provide orientation in difficult circumstances and a magnifier that can help me to search for other possibilities when all my knowledge and resources seems be insufficient.

The River That Opens the Road

We are approaching the destination, but I feel higher than ever beyond the more distant clouds, because now I can finally see the bigger picture and realize that those images and metaphors I cultivated most frequently during the last hours are not totally odd and inconsistent. It was not by mistake or chance that I figure myself navigating the sea once and sailing along a river another time. I was merely not aware that those metaphors depicted different scenarios, two distinctive kinds of journey and exploration. The components of my metaphoric navigation are actually two: navigating *among others* and *within myself*. There is the sea where I cooperate and I build with others, and the freshwater where I get myself ready to face the big waves of the ocean. Two unique areas in constant communication are merging into each other; two domains that I explored on this journey using different symbols without even realizing it. It is good I did not analyze too much, and allowed myself to move further on this journey. What could appear initially like nonsense talking about crew, captains, river, sea, harbors and lakes led to something interesting.

Here, up in the sky, as I look down to see the islands becoming bigger, I realize something I was not conscious before: my navigation across the sea was where I invested the most and I can admit that it has been extensive and fruitful. Unlike my internal sailing along rivers and lakes, the research I do to go to sea has became a fulltime activity that starts before my departure and does not end at my return. I don't wait anymore for understanding and lucidity to happen, but carefully look for them. I realize now that in this vast sea I am exploring, I have what is needed to keep progressing, and building proficiency. Actually, it is a river that stopped me the longer. It is the "inner navigation" where all these years I advanced less and struggled the most. I had my regular supervision and therapy, but my internal preparation never became a regular exercise as is the case with all the study, writing and consultation when I want to get ready for a new project. Is there an athlete who focuses merely on training, while forgetting the mental preparation, the discipline in habits, and nutrition? No way, I cannot believe I took this part of my work as complementary, because the two kinds of navigation are equally important, nourishing, and they complete each other. Unlike a *proper* researcher and explorer, in my internal work I lacked in pro-activity, mindset and tools. I was full of good intentions and wandered a lot along the internal pathway, making several attempts, but to begin with I missed completely the *propaedeutic* component. As an individual and especially as a professional, I cannot leave the discoveries of the internal realm to chance. There is so much work to do, and I realize that I have to define my internal MAP to purposefully move forward.

I should approach matters as a proper researcher, starting by constantly applying the four *pro* steps, and list the reference points I have already uncovered. I know for instance that Primo and my guidebook are my companions in everything I do. For this reason, I need to know them better, not just to get along but to access a wider knowledge based and abilities and expand my possibilities in all situations. I am aware I have to look for verticality, take off regularly and enjoy the navigation in *diagonal* with the process and proceed modality. I also discovered another thing: everything should be flavored with playfulness. I have to remind myself to play: play with ideas, play with expressive modalities, and most importantly play my own new scripts. Those might sound like little discoveries, but they make me feel good and I want to celebrate reading another part of one of my favorite poems, the *Song of the Open Road* by Walt Whitman (Poetry Foundation 2021a):

> Afoot and light-hearted I take to the open road,
> Healthy, free, the world before me,
> The long brown path before me leading wherever I choose.
>
> Henceforth I ask not good-fortune, I myself am good-fortune,
> Henceforth I whimper no more, postpone no more, need nothing,
> Done with indoor complaints, libraries, querulous criticisms,
> Strong and content I travel the open road.

I like this poem because is a conquest, the result of an internal journey and, at the same time, the beginning of a new one. Somehow I feel the same with my search for internal reference points. In a way it is a path I have just started, even though it took me a long way to get here. Like the poet, I also carried my burden along the way, something that I can't get rid of as any part of my story, but here I realized that what I thought was limiting my possibilities "keeping me along the coast," is actually the reason for my strength and the courage to navigate the entire hydrography. An extra sparkle of understanding and a few lines added to my own story changed everything. The luggage of my experiences that I wanted to lose or lighten at times, here beyond the clouds, became the springboard for a new open road. This is the road of personal and professional possibilities where I can progress and be more productive. I already see something exciting in this new space of possibilities.

It is the image (Figure 5) I drew some minutes ago. Looking at it with different eyes I can perceive something emerging. It is a rudder! A symbol that represents being in control and allows direction for external and internal explorations and learning. I found my treasure today with this, because I can use it as a reminder, a goal to keep in mind and also a tool to promote self-awareness.

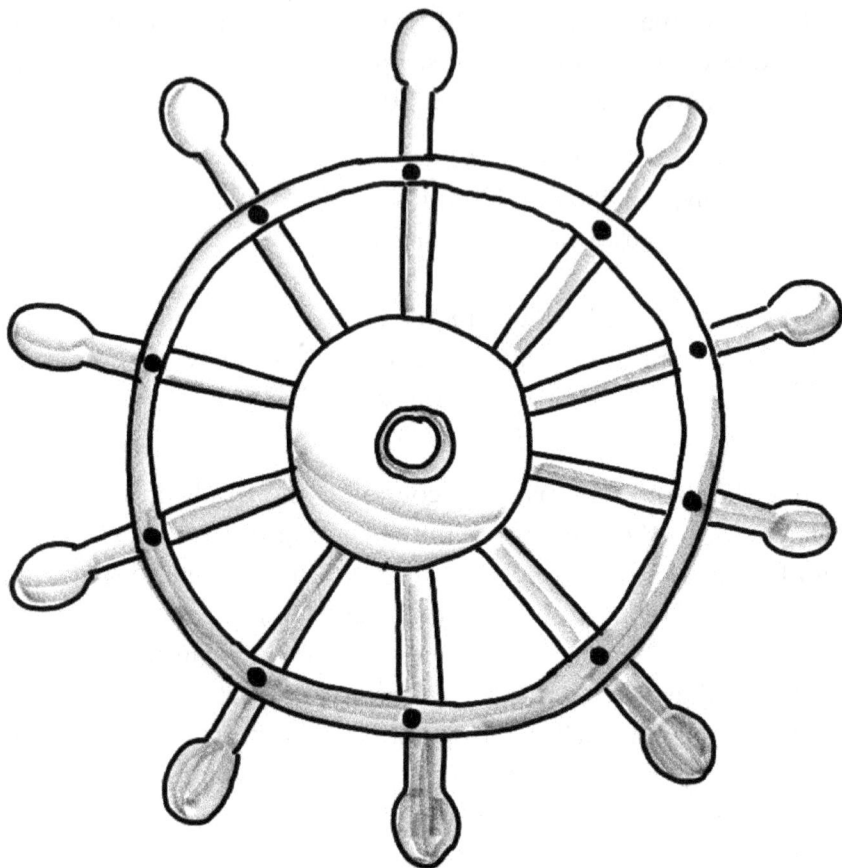

Fig. 11. A ship's wheel (controls the rudder).

I can already imagine a couple of activities for my students and clients based on it. I will call them "The revealing rudder," parts I and II. Navigating is never the same and it can be very hard, because there are so many conditions that affect the sailing and the feeling of being in control, as much as there are in every ability and item of knowledge we use (or could use) to keep us out of danger and to reach our destination.

In the first part of the activity, I imagine inviting them to draw a rudder in the middle of a piece of paper and then to divide it in three parts. The lower one around the rudder represents the water and all the elements that might jeopardize navigation and the feeling of being in charge. As in the actual sailing, where there are dangers underneath the water, waves that shock the vessel and a powerful stream to manage, also in the metaphorical navigation there are a number of challenges that can be represented by drawing. As for the other parts of the representation, each of these items can be further analyzed and described in detail, individually or in groups.

In the upper part of the paper, there is the world outside the water. This second part portrays the destination and possible inter-mediate goals symbolized by islands or any other shape that makes sense to the individual. In this section, the trainee or client can also include the factors that might obstruct a clear vision of the destination in the same way as when there is rainfall or a storm interfering with vision.

The third and last section is the one enclosed within the rudder, where we can find all the resources and abilities we use to sail and to remain in charge of the boat. Here we can insert everything and everyone that helps us to keep or regain control, to face different challenges, what we use to reach clarity for our direction and any other element that is supportive in reaching our destination. Once all three parts and elements are drawn, I will invite the group to discuss the most significant elements of the drawing in pairs, then to give it a title and to share it with the group.

Another application also comes to my mind, or part II of the activity, which could fit particularly for my students, and considers all the different *pros* of our rudder (those represented in Table 1). Each component should be drawn according to our perception. We can draw on the same sheet of paper or another one, using different sizes or shapes, the entity of our investment, or the results we achieved for each *pro*. We could also decide to add specific descrip-tions or considerations inside the different elements. The final creation would provide an overview of the work we have done as professionals and be a useful guide for reflections on future actions. Also in this case, I find it useful to share verbally what was drawn.

I am happy that at the end of this journey I can count on one more resource, also because it can apply perfectly to crisis work. In critical circumstances, professionals might need to provide guidance and sustain other people's navigation but, most of all, the rudder depicts the essence of the entire intervention: supporting individuals and communities in gaining awareness and acquiring the resources to be in charge of their own boat and to access the open sea of possibilities.

Conclusion ~ Landing

We are going to land soon. I did not let my work slide, in fact I slept just after finishing what I had planned. I think I performed an important step here: been a professional, not a procrastinator. I fed the wolf[18] of learning from the experience. I fought the urge to give up[19] and kept going.

Focus, clarity, integration and a new course of action prevailed. I understood I needed to write to clarify my thoughts and organize my work, and I resisted the temptation to think, "I will do it one day!" Now, I have completed a lot of work in preparation for the forthcoming days, a good structure for my book, and I added new and unexpected lines to my personal narrative.

We have landed! People are applauding the captain. Soon I will meet my new colleagues. Let me check: I have my MAP, some internal reference points, clear terms for my work, a self-care program to follow, and a plan "B" with a shorter self-care routine in case of more hectic days. I also have set the program for when I will be back, including making space and time to reflect and write, supervision and so on. Great, I have everything.

---

[18] This sentence refers to the story known as the *Grandfather Tell*. The origin is most probably a Cherokee legend that tells about a grandfather using a metaphor of two wolves fighting within him to explain his inner conflicts to his grandson. When his grandson asks which wolf wins, the grandfather answers, whichever he chooses to feed (Firstpeople.us. 2019).

[19] Herbert Nitsch is the world record holder for free diving. In 2012 he spoke to the BBC World Service and said "Only the time you have the urge to breathe and fight against it, that's the time you are actually training" (BBC World Service 2019).

Of course, we will never be bulletproof; Brené Brown[20] (2002) is right. We are vulnerable and imperfect, and waiting for perfection should not be a justification for not taking action. Particularly in this field, being aware that we are all vulnerable offers good reasons to pay attention to our propaedeutics.

In a few minutes, I will be in a crowded bus and then in a crowded hangar; for several hours this will be the last calm moment. I want to use this time to write a reminder for myself:

Everything looks ready now but, once on the deck of the new vessel, everything will be less familiar in so many ways: this whole experience will be different and you will be different. So let go of the expectations built in other places, be kind to yourself and be open to embrace it all.

---

[20] Brené Brown is the author of *Daring Greatly*. In the introduction of her book she writes: "When we spend our lives waiting until we're perfect or bulletproof before we walk into the arena, we ultimately sacrifice relationships and opportunities that may not be recoverable, we squander our precious time, and we turn our backs on our gifts, those unique contributions that only we can make. Perfect and bulletproof are seductive, but they don't exist in the human experience" (Brown 2012).

References

American Psychological Association (2020) *APA dictionary of psychology*, available: https://dictionary.apa.org/respect [accessed 10 January 2020].

ATLAS.ti - Qualitative Data Analysis (2014) *Wall, Sarah - Autoethnography: possibility and controversy*, available: https://www.youtube.com/watch?v=pEWF0SV9F_s [accessed 29 November 2019].

BBC World Service (2019) *Outlook - The deepest man on earth - BBC Sounds*, available: https://www.bbc.co.uk/sounds/play/w3csz386 [accessed 10 January 2020].

Bochner, A.P. & Riggs, N.A. (2014) 'Practicing narrative inquiry', in Leavy, P. (ed.) *The Oxford handbook of qualitative research*, Oxford University Press, 195-222.

Bochner, A.P. (2016) *Coming to narrative: A personal history of paradigm change in the human sciences*, Walnut Creek, CA: Left Coast Press, Inc.

Bodenoch, B. (2008) *Being a brain-wise therapist: A practical guide to interpersonal neurobiology*, NY: WW Norton & Company, Kindle edition.

Brooks, R. (2000) *Education and "charismatic" adults: To touch a student's heart and mind*, available:

https://www.drrobertbrooks.com/wp2/wp-content/uploads/2000/09/Education-and-Charismatic-Adults-To-Touch-a-Students-Heart-and-Mind.pdf [accessed 8 December 2019].

Brooks, R. & Goldstein, S. (2015) 'The power of mindsets. Guideposts for a resilience-based treatment approach', in D.A., Crenshaw, R., Brooks & S., Goldstein (eds.) *Play therapy interventions to enhance resilience*, New York: Guilford Press, 168-193.

Brown, B. (2012) *Daring greatly: How the courage to be vulnerable transforms the way we live, love, parent, and lead*, New York, NY: Gotham Books, Kindle edition.

Cassina, I. (2020) *The magic home. A displaced boy finds a way to feel better*, Ann Arbor, MI: Loving Healing Press.

Cassina, I. (2020) *Expressive arts research and philosophy*, unpublished essay (CAGS), Switzerland: European Graduate School.

Cohen, A. (1990) *Joy is my compass: Taking the risk to follow your bliss*, Dolphin Communications Company, Kindle edition.

Chang, H. (2007), "Autoethnography: Raising Cultural Consciousness of Self and Others", Walford, G. (Ed.) *Methodological Developments in Ethnography (Studies in Educational Ethnography, Vol. 12)*, Emerald Group Publishing Limited, Bingley, pp. 207-221. https://doi.org/10.1016/S1529-210X(06)12012-4

Cozolino, L. (2016) "Why therapy works," *The Neuropsychotherapist*, 4(1), 7-16.

Damasio, A. (1999) *The feeling of what happens. Body and emotions in the making of consciousness*, San Diego, CA: Harvest Book Harcourt, Inc.

Dilts, R. (1996) *Visionary leadership skills. Creating a world to which people want to belong*, Meta Publications, Capitola, Ca.

Drewes, A.A. & Schaefer, C.E. (2014) "Introduction: How play therapy causes therapeutic changes," in C.E., Schaefer & A.A., Drewes (eds.) *The therapeutic powers of play*, New Jersey: Wiley, 1-7.

Ellis, C. (2004) *The Etnographic I. A methodological novel about autoetnography*, Walnut Creek, CA: Altamira Press.

Firstpeople.us (2019) *Two wolves a Cherokee legend*, available: https://www.firstpeople.us/FP-Html-Legends/TwoWolves-Cherokee.html [accessed 11 July 2019].

Flytenewmedia (2020) *Nurturing resilience in yourself and your team during a crisis with Dr Robert Brooks*, available:

https://www.youtube.com/watch?v=XgJHMEpHGBE&t=4s [accessed 20 April 2020].

ICQM - Israeli Center for Qualitative Research of People and Societies, Ben-Gurion University of the Negev (2015) *Autoethnography in qualitative inquiry - Professor Carolyn Ellis and Professor Arthur Bochner*, available: https://www.youtube.com/watch?v=FKZ-wuJ_vnQ [accessed 26 November 2019].

Inter-Agency Standing Committee (2007) *IASC guidelines on mental health and psychosocial support in emergency settings*, Geneva: IASC, available: http://www.humanitarianinfo.org/iasc/content/products [accessed 9 May 2014].

Ludy-Dobson, C.R. & Perry, B.D. (2010) "The role of healthy interaction in buffering the impact of childhood trauma," in E., Gil (ed.) *Working with children to heal interpersonal trauma: The power of play*, New York: Guilford Press, 26-43.

Katz, M. (1981) "Isolation fuels Hagler's intent," *New York Times*, 20 Apr, available: https://www.nytimes.com/1981/01/16/sports/isolation-fuels-hagler-s-intent.html [accessed 20 September 2021].

Kestly, T. (2014) *The interpersonal neurobiology of play: Brain-building interventions for emotional well-being*, New York, NY: Norton.

Kestly, T. (2016) "Presence and play: Why mindfulness matters," *International Journal of Play Therapy*, 25(1), 14-23.

Masten, A.S. (2001) "Ordinary magic: Resilience processes in development," *American Psychologist*, 56, 227-238.

Masters, E.L. (2000) *Spoon River Anthology*, Penn State Electronic Classics Series Publication.

McGilchrist, I. (2012) *The master and his emissary: The divided brain and the making of the Western world*, London: Yale UP, Kindle edition.

McGilchrist, I. (2019) *The master and his emissary: The divided brain and the making of the Western world*, new expanded edition, New Haven and London: Yale University Press.

Mochi, C. (2009) "Trauma repetition: intervention in psychological safe places," *Eastern Journal of Psychiatry*, 12, 73-80.

Mochi, C. (2017) *Play therapy in developing/emerging countries* and *Using play therapy in post disaster scenario*, conferences presented at the Australasia Pacific Play Therapy Association APPTA Annual Conference, Sydney, 14 August 2017.

Mochi, C. & VanFleet, R. (2009) "Roles play therapist play. Post disaster engagement and empowerment of survivors," *Play Therapy Magazine*, 4(4), 16-18.

Mochi, C. & Cassina, I. (2018) *Play Therapy around the globe: International crisis work with children*, training presented at Northwest Center for Play Therapy Studies Summer Institute, George Fox University, Portland, 6 June 2018.

Mochi, C. & Cassina, I. (2020) *International crisis: The potential of play therapy and expressive arts modalities*, webinar presented for Inspirees Institute and International Association of Creative Arts Somatic Education, 23 March 2020.

Naiaretti, C., Sagramoso, A. & Solaro del Borgo, M.A. (2006) *Strumenti operativi per progetti di cooperazione allo sviluppo*, 2nd edn., Lugano: Federazione delle ONG della Svizzera Italiana (FOSIT).

Panksepp, J. & Biven, L. (2012) *The archaeology of mind: Neuroevolutionary origins of human emotions*, New York, NY: Norton.

Perry, B.D. (1997) "Incubated terror: The neurodevelopmental factors in the cycle of violence," in J. D. Osofsky (ed.) *Children in a violent society*, New York: Guilford press, 124-149.

Perry, B.D. (2013) *Introduction to the neurosequential model of therapeutics (NMT)*, available:
https://www.thenationalcouncil.org/wp-

content/uploads/2012/11/Bruce-Perry-Slides.pdf?daf=375ateTbd56 [accessed 21 July 2021].

Perry, B.D. (2020) "Interview on: Childhood trauma," *Being Well with Dr. Rick Hanson*, available: https://www.rickhanson.net/being-well-podcast-childhood-trauma-with-dr-bruce-perry/ [accessed 7 March 2021].

Poetry Foundation (2021a) *Song of the open road*, available: https://www.poetryfoundation.org/poems/48859/song-of-the-open-road [accessed 30 September 2021].

Poetry Foundation (2021b) *The road not taken*, available: https://www.poetryfoundation.org/poems/44272/the-road-not-taken [accessed 5 August 2021].

Porges, S. (2011) *The polyvagal theory: Neurophysiological foundations of emotions, attachment, communication, and self-regulation*, New York, NY: Norton.

Schaefer, C.E. (1993) "What is play and what is it therapeutic?" in C.E. Schaefer (ed.) *The therapeutic power of play*, Northwale, N.J.: Jason Aronson, 1-15.

Schaefer, C.E. & Drewes, A.A. (eds.) (2014) *The therapeutic powers of play*, New Jersey: Wiley.

Siegel, D. & Bryson, T.D. (2016) *No drama discipline workbook*, New York: Bantam.

SMCBGSU - School of Media and Communication, Bowling Green State University (2016) *The rise of autoethnography: Stretching boundaries, fashioning identities, healing wounds*, available: https://www.youtube.com/watch?v=X3EJfPN9sIg [accessed 21 November 2019].

ThougthCo (2019) *Is "first do no harm" part of the Hippocratic oath?*, available: https://www.thoughtco.com/first-do-no-harm-hippocratic-oath-118780 [accessed 9 August 2019].

United Nations Development Programme (2016) *Human development report 2016*, available: http://hdr.undp.org/sites/default/files/2016_human_development_report.pdf [accessed 8 July 2017].

United Nations High Commissioner for Refugees (2015) *Emergency handbook*, available: https://emergency.unhcr.org/entry/43085/collective-centre-coordination-and-management?fbclid=IwAR2hpzZ6dESLl_Duj1yXrUcl19f0Ohq_C3efJ9kl_A31E_q93T5X4OabSm0 [accessed 9 January 2020].

van der Kolk, B. (2000) *Posttraumatic stress disorder and the nature of trauma. Dialogues in clinical neuroscience*, 2(1), 7-22.

van der Kolk, B. (2001) 'The assessment and treatment of complex PTSD', in R., Yehuda (ed.) *Treating trauma survivors with PTSD*, Washington, DC: American Psychiatric Publishing, Inc., 127-156.

VanFleet, R. (2012) *A parent's handbook of filial therapy: Building strong families with play*, 2nd edn., Boiling Springs, PA: Play Therapy Press.

VanFleet, R. & Mochi, C. (2015) Enhancing resilience through play therapy with child and family survivors of mass trauma, in D.A., Crenshaw, R. Brooks & S. Goldstein (eds.) *Play therapy interventions to enhance resilience*, New York: Guilford Press, 168-193.

Vygotskii, L.S., & Cole, M. (1978). *Mind in society: The development of higher psychological processes*. Cambridge: Harvard University Press.

Wikipedia (2020) *Propaedeutics*, available: https://en.wikipedia.org/wiki/Propaedeutics[accessed 9 January 2020].

Vygotsky, L.S. (1978) *Mind in society: The development of higher psychological processes*, Cambridge, MA: Harvard University Press

About the Author

Looking back on my own educational journey, I realize that I had many ups and downs. As an enthusiastic Montessori-inspired kindergartner, I remember an enormous curiosity about the trees we tended and climbed and the garden that was so full of possibilities. I loved exploring, growing, and inventing. I remember friends, the games we played together and even some tasty foods, but not the time when I learned to read and write. It wasn't until my senior year of kindergarten that I have any memory of a strictly didactic experience as I wrote a few words in English. At the time, I was unaware of how much less interesting my experience would be at school, with the exception of soccer games.

The first day of elementary school, I felt trapped at my desk. The trees were no longer a place of conversation, but remained in the background. Engaging and spontaneous learning was already a distant memory. It was a real joy that same day to see my brother climbing over the school wall and coming in from the garden to greet me! When everyone had left, the teacher invited us to draw something, and there he was, cheering me on. *How did he know I needed support so badly?* I don't remember much else about that day but, within those walls and the soccer field, I met the best friends that I still hold dear.

From a very young age, I was in love with books that told of faraway places, legends, and the lives of animals, and yet in school, we started over with the alphabet. While I was leaving something on the way, I was learning that to go on I could put less effort as possible. Because of this and a bit of a rebellious spirit, I was among the few in my entire school to have to repeat a year in seventh grade. All my dear friends were moving on and only thanks to the determination of my mother did I avoid expulsion from school. In the Roman suburbs where we lived, that private school was considered high-profile, and I believe that enrolling there had been quite an effort for my parents. I had failed them, I had let them down and I felt I wasn't worth enough for not being able to get ahead and keep up with the others.

I couldn't have known then that these intimate experiences of disappointment, guilt and feeling of being not worth are more common than I thought. Exactly within a year, with the passing of my brother in a motorcycle accident right in front of that school, I learned that what seemed like a tragedy to me was actually nothing. My being constantly late had prevented me from witnessing the accident. That afternoon I was supposed to play the final game of the soccer championship at that same school. This year, everything had changed. I understood many things and, among them, that I would have continued to learn even the things that didn't interest me. I would have followed in my brother's footsteps and started studying at the School of Commerce, which he could not finish.

The passion for my studies came with last years of secondary school and increased further with the thesis in Clinical Psychology while I was investigating how the integration of mind and body could be achieved through the study and practice of Qi Gong. Apart from this, my years at university had been quite dull without opportunities to practice. *How is it conceivable that one can learn only by reading and replicating contents?* What I was learning at school did not enrich me as a person, and what I was learning as a person was added no value to my studies and my qualities as a student. I was in my twenties and I had the urge to learn, explore, apply and face challenges. Instead, I was tied up to a chair studying ten months out of the year. The reasoning of how our educational path is structured is still obscure to me, but I exercised a lot of discipline and eventually I earned a degree and a professional license.

I became a doctor in Clinical and Community Psychology and yet the most formative experiences of those years were the extra-curricular ones organized by the Italian government and myself. As an alternative to the military, I did my community service in a home for minors where I ended up being in charge. Nevertheless, I was twenty-two years old and too immature to maintain that huge responsibility. After twenty intense and beautiful months, I resumed my path. Another enriching experience was the sabbatical time I took during university. According to the results of my exams, I was able to take up to three months at a time to travel the world alone. With the money earned from various jobs, I traveled all over Europe and then in North Africa, Middle East and Asia. I saw and learned a lot and started to consolidate the habit of interacting with people from different cultures and balancing exploration, family and studies.

In distant and remote contexts, I felt more inspired, passionate, and curious. I reached a deeper level of thought and awareness, and I also practiced a broader and more complete repertoire of skills and behaviors. It is fascinating to think that the desert, the ocean and trekking in the Himalayas were my improving ingredients and growth factors. As I write these lines, I realize that I have benefited from slowing down and detaching from my daily life. In moments of solitude staring at the sky and vast horizons, instead of getting lost, I was finding myself. By wandering around, I was probably reclaiming some parts of myself and resuming learning in a natural and passionate way, as we did in kindergarten. On the contrary, the pile of theories to memorize and the professional scenarios ahead of me seemed to lead me exactly in the opposite direction.

A few months after I discussed my thesis, during a long swim in the Caribbean Sea, I was gloating at the idea of having turned down an unlikely position at the university as "almost-assistant to the vice professor". In disbelief, I stopped in the water and congratulated myself for not having accepted what seemed to be not only an unpaid position, but also one with limited opportunities. I knew then that the vacation would be over and once I returned home I would be lucky to accept a job that I did not like. Nevertheless, I felt strong and content because I was aware that, at that point, I would never stop aspiring to something that would motivate me deeply and make really sense to me. I wanted something I could commit all of myself and provide me opportunities to grow as a person.

This something took the form of Emergency Psychology and disaster interventions. I think the big motivating factor back then was to provide support to people at the moment when it was needed most. I felt there was great value in being present in circumstances in which even a small gesture could be significant to people. I also thought that in emergencies there was more scope for action than in the careers that lay ahead of me. After qualification, I worked for a few years in some psychosocial rehabilitation and drug addiction projects. I learned a lot and did my best even though I was always looking for opportunities to learn more about trauma and emergency interventions. I participated in a two-year training in Emergency Psychology and took multiple other training such as EMDR level I and II, Critical Incident Stress Debriefing, and even a workshop on Hostage Negotiation.

At the time, there weren't a lot of international programs that included mental health professionals. I tried very hard to succeed and after a short Peacekeeping experience I started working on a couple of projects in the Balkans. After that, I worked on four different projects in Iran, and then other projects in Lebanon, Pakistan, Sri Lanka, Palestine and Haiti. I cooperated internationally with mid-sized and large humanitarian organizations for almost a decade. I was lucky in that period because I tried to learn from my mistakes and my limits. Professionally, I was still not very solid in specialized treatments, but then I discovered Play Therapy during my work in Iran.

After the earthquake in Bam, I was hired to set up a clinic for the most difficult cases. I was supposed to be one of the experts to whom refer difficult situations, but the play spaces managed by some local psychiatrists seemed to do a much better job with children and youth. They were using the power of play to help the young survivors to feel better and overcome trauma. This was a great lesson that reminded me to be open, flexible, and humble. In the Iranian desert I took my first Play Therapy training and, from that moment, I started to combine intensive studies in Play Therapy around the world and kept working in post-disaster and conflict areas. There were very intense years, but I could balance quality time with my family and the commitment in extending my abilities to be supportive in all aspects of crisis interventions, from psychological first aid to the most specialized treatment.

I always considered the crisis intervention like a dialogue more than a speech. The moment I realized that the space for co-discussion and co-creation of projects and programs was too limited, I decided not to renew my work contract with a certain organization. I noticed that, in many contexts, what counts is what you say you do, and less the quality of the process and the long-term results. At the end of my term in Haiti, for example, an architect took my place and this confirmed how right I was. I was angry and frustrated, but I had a moment of enjoyment when my replacement was appointed since I could send to the entire staff an article I wrote with Risë VanFleet that was published that very day about the role of mental health professionals in disasters! For several years, I wrote as an emotional release when I felt it was the only way to cope with the situation. With time, and most of all traveling "beyond the clouds", writing became a source of research and understanding that opened new unexpected possibilities.

After my work in Haiti, I found out that the most difficult location where to start a project was five hundred meters from my parents' home. The first time I applied for a location was to set up a psychosocial centre in a big public housing complex, the local administration replied that "my proposal was very interesting, but unfortunately I had no political affiliation". I did not need any political affiliation when I founded the Italian Association for Play Therapy (APTI) in 2009. I had experienced the immense value of Play Therapy and I wanted to promote quality training, supervision and practice. During my attempts to promote different projects in my home country, I kept studying with some of the most renown Play Therapists in the world. A few years after, I co-founded with my life partner the International Academy for Play Therapy studies and Psychosocial Projects (INA) in Switzerland.

It was not easy for our small Association to launch high level courses for specialized professionals and psychosocial programs, but with time we had the opportunity to present training and conferences internationally in over twenty different countries and to run long term projects in Italy, Switzerland, Nigeria and India. The more time passes, the more I am able to enjoy the freedom to develop tailor-made activities and to suffer from as few limitations as possible in the process. Structuring high profile courses and projects and making them available even in the most remote places of the world motivates me a lot. The same goes for the hard work of refining everything I am learning and accumulating in the process.

Many years have passed, but it is still not crystal clear to me why I chose this path that has marked almost half of my life. The reason for choosing a job in exhausting contexts in which you are in full-time contact with suffering is hard to fathom. So it is to offer the intangible in times when people have lost everything! What motivates one to engage in such an activity? This choice cannot be completely conscious. I would have to research and delve deeper to learn more. With time, however, I became aware I have gained other certainties.

I know that the vast majority of the teachers I had in the early years had no practical experience, their teaching was purely theoretical and as such dangerous. Since my first crisis and post-disaster interventions in Italy, I realized that their preaching of prepackaged interventions could never work, at least not for the survivors' wellbeing. On the contrary, these contexts require professionals to stop and understand first. In these years, I understood that before techniques and protocols comes human contact. Everything a professional learns as technician *and* as individual matters. I am also certain that these experiences can be very tough. In fact, while pushing the professional to seek flexibility, breadth of vision and repertoire of actions on the one hand, on the other hand they affect the individual in his or her innermost self in the exact opposite direction.

I do not know why I went along this path, but I feel that I made the right choice. So far, I spent almost three thousand days in the field with the great opportunity to work in different contexts and cultures with individuals, families, and entire communities. I met remarkable people and had the joy to see many of them taking back charge of their lives. Assisting these strenuous journeys had a massive impact on me, it motivated me to improve and research in different directions. This book is a relevant part of this path.

Index

The Magic Home: A Displaced Boy Finds a Way to Feel Better

The Magic Home is a story for those who believe in magic, to turn fear into bravery and let fantasies run wild! This is a tale of a little boy that lives with his family, plays happily in the courtyard with his brother, sister, a brown dog and a fluffy white rabbit, and cannot wait to start school. Suddenly he has to leave for an unpredictable journey...

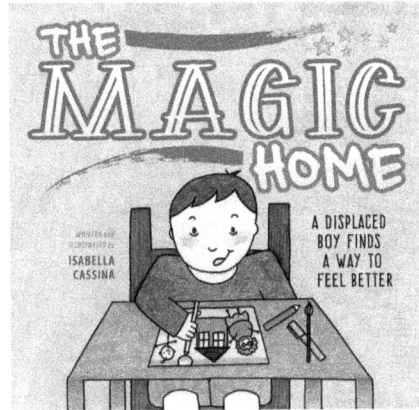

The Magic Home offers psycho-educational support for children, parents and childhood professionals who are assisting children through the difficult transition of displacement. The author presents a guide for caregivers grounded in the principles of Play Therapy that allows children to be engaged in a dynamic and engaging process based on their capacities and the objectives defined by a caring adult. The book is ideal for easy reading with individuals and groups, and the suggested activities can be used between parent and child, at school, in a healthcare agency or any other place where children spend time.

"*The Magic Home* is an endearing and enduring story of a child's journey to deal with unimaginable feelings of sadness, loss and displacement. This touching story teaches us how to tap into the child's resilience using the healing power of play and expressive arts. *The Magic Home* is a must-have book for child clinicians, caregivers and child professionals to use with children displaced from their homes, regardless of the situation."
-- Athena A. Drewes, PsyD, MA, RPT-S, founder and president emeritus of the New York Association for Play Therapy.

"*The Magic Home* is a comforting story about a little boy who loses all that is familiar and faces many uncertainties in his new life until he meets Ina, who helps him feel that he is not alone. This gently told story and sweet illustrations offer children who have faced disruptions in their families a sense of control over their circumstances and hope for a brighter future."
-- Sue Bratton, PhD, LPC-S, RPT-S, director emerita, Center for Play Therapy at University of North Texas

"*The Magic Home* takes us on a journey that is dealing with loss, adjustment and, most importantly, feelings. This book helps adults help children with big feelings that are hard to understand. The added suggestions on how to use the book and reusable figures are a valuable addition. A delightful and helpful book that helps us all know we have a magic home. "
-- Linda E. Homeyer, PhD, LPCS, RPT-S, distinguished professor emerita and past president of the Association for Play Therapy (APT) board of directors.

paperback * hardcover * eBook *audiobook

From Loving Healing Press
www.LHPress.com

www.ingramcontent.com/pod-product-compliance
Lightning Source LLC
Chambersburg PA
CBHW070407200326
41518CB00011B/2097